"Colleen Carney has taken the complex field of adolescent sleep and circadian science research, and crafted its most supported findings into an easy-to-read book filled with useful information that can be quickly learned and utilized to improve sleep health. The use of case studies, hands-on activities, and step-by-step instructions make this book an excellent resource for teens, parents, and providers to help address many of the sleep problems and related obstacles that are unique to today's teens."

—**Allison K. Wilkerson, PhD**, licensed psychologist, and assistant professor at Medical University of South Carolina

"Sleep affects everyone across the age range, but each age group has their own unique sleep difficulties. Colleen Carney has put together the ideal book for teens and their families, physicians, and support network to understand, identify, and address the idiosyncrasies of teen sleep. Many teens and their families can benefit from this book, which lays out a clear plan and offers evidence-based tips any teen can follow to improve their sleep."

—**Katherine Marczyk Organek, PhD**, pediatric sleep psychologist at Cook Children's Medical Center

"Teens are sadly not exempt from sleep problems, and insomnia is an ever-growing issue in this population. Colleen Carney's book is a valuable resource for adolescents and their parents, helping all members at home achieve a better night's sleep. A practical, straight-forward, and scientifically backed approach to targeting insomnia, *Goodnight Mind for Teens* will also be of great use to the vast majority of teachers, therapists, and pediatricians who work with this population. Good sleep habits should be taught early on, and Carney's book lays a fantastic groundwork for a lifetime of healthy sleep."

> —**Shelby F. Harris, PsyD**, author of *The Women's Guide to Overcoming Insomnia*, and clinical associate professor of neurology at the Albert Einstein College of Medicine

"This engaging book is a must-read for teenagers who have difficulty sleeping. Problems with sleep during the teenage years are common, and can lead to difficulties with learning, attention, memory, and many other daytime consequences. Colleen Carney speaks directly to teens with her succinct writing style and clear approach to managing insomnia. The book includes education about sleep and evidence-based treatment suggestions, as well as clear summaries and 'plans for the week' in every chapter. Teenagers, parents, and anyone who works with teens will benefit from reading this book, which will empower teens to improve their own sleep."

> —**Shelly Weiss, MD, FRCPC**, pediatric neurologist, professor, and faculty of medicine at the University of Toronto; author of *Better Sleep for Your Baby and Child*; and past president of the Canadian Sleep Society

the *i* n s t a n t h e l p
s o l u t i o n s   s e r i e s

Young people today need mental health resources more than ever. That's why New Harbinger created the **Instant Help Solutions Series** especially for teens. Written by leading psychologists, physicians, and professionals, these evidence-based self-help books offer practical tips and strategies for dealing with a variety of mental health issues and life challenges teens face, such as depression, anxiety, bullying, eating disorders, trauma, and self-esteem problems.

Studies have shown that young people who learn healthy coping skills early on are better able to navigate problems later in life. Engaging and easy-to-use, these books provide teens with the tools they need to thrive—at home, at school, and on into adulthood.

This series is part of the **New Harbinger Instant Help Books** imprint, founded by renowned child psychologist Lawrence Shapiro. For a complete list of books in this series, visit newharbinger.com.

goodnight mind for teens

skills to help you quiet noisy thoughts & get the sleep you need

COLLEEN E. CARNEY, PhD

Instant Help Books
An Imprint of New Harbinger Publications, Inc.

Publisher's Note

Distributed in Canada by Raincoast Books

Copyright © 2020 by Colleen E. Carney
    Instant Help Books
    An imprint of New Harbinger Publications, Inc.
    5674 Shattuck Avenue
    Oakland, CA 94609
    www.newharbinger.com

Cover design by Amy Shoup; Acquired by Jess O'Brien; Edited by Ken Knabb

Library of Congress Cataloging-in-Publication Data

Names: Carney, Colleen, author.
Title: Goodnight mind for teens : skills to help you quiet noisy thoughts and get the sleep you need / Colleen E. Carney.
Description: Oakland : Instant Help Books, an imprint of New Harbinger Publications, Inc., [2020] | Series: The instant help solutions series | Audience: Ages 14-18
Identifiers: LCCN 2019056571 (print) | LCCN 2019056572 (ebook) | ISBN 9781684034383 (paperback) | ISBN 9781684034390 (pdf) | ISBN 9781684034406 (epub)
Subjects: LCSH: Insomnia--Treatment. | Sleep disorders in adolescence--Treatment. | Affective disorders--Treatment. | Cognitive therapy.
Classification: LCC RC548 .C3644 2020 (print) | LCC RC548 (ebook) | DDC 616.8/498--dc23
LC record available at https://lccn.loc.gov/2019056571
LC ebook record available at https://lccn.loc.gov/2019056572

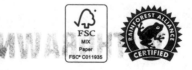

Printed in the United States of America

22 21 20

10 9 8 7 6 5 4 3 2 1   First Printing

Contents

Using This Book

Unfortunately, many teens and young adults complain that they have sleep problems and that nothing seems to help. I noticed that much of what was available for teens was actually written for kids or for adults. But teens' sleep problems are unique. So I decided to write a book that specifically addresses those problems.

- Do you have difficulty with not being able to fall asleep quickly?

- Do you wake up in the middle of the night and find it difficult to return to sleep quickly?

- Do you fall asleep during the day?

- Do you feel like you need to sleep for long periods on the weekends?

If you answered yes to any or all of these questions, there are things that you can do to feel better!

HELP IS ON THE WAY

If you are reading this book, you are probably one of the many teens struggling with sleep or with feeling tired. You are not alone. There are many reasons to want to sleep better, including feeling better and improving your health. I have designed this book so that the tips in the chapters correspond to the most common sleep-related problems faced by teens. The tips within each chapter are specific, tailored to your sleep information from a sleep tracking form you complete, and the goals you set to improve your sleep are entirely determined by you.

We have very effective treatments for insomnia for kids and adults. However, teens face unique sleep problems that limit their ability to use child-focused sleep resources. Treatments for children focus on parents strictly controlling bedtimes and wake times, but adolescence is a time when teens are supposed to be learning to be more independent. Treatments for adults do not focus on the body-clock problems created by sex hormones during puberty, or on the pattern of oversleeping on the weekends. Teens need their own treatment adapted from state-of-the-art sleep medicine research. This treatment is based on cognitive behavioral therapy (CBT) and it has been shown to be effective in young adults. CBT is an approach that assumes that changing your thoughts and behaviors can change the way you feel and can help with health-related problems. Of course, CBT may not be for everyone. Other options include medications that may be offered by your doctor. However, most experts agree that not enough is known about the safety and long-term effects of sleeping medications, and that CBT is usually a preferable frontline treatment. This means that CBT should be offered to teens first.

Most teens say they prefer to direct their own treatment. This is referred to as "self-management." As a result, there has been a trend to provide CBT tools to teens, but in a way that allows you to choose what strategies to use and what goals to set. Self-management empowers you to set goals that you know you can achieve. Achieving success in your goals and experiencing the benefits makes you feel more confident to make further changes. Many teens say they are frustrated that they are told to follow a specific schedule that results in them lying awake unable to sleep, and then they are criticized when they are unable to get out of bed in the morning at the time they are "supposed" to get up. This creates a cycle of conflict between parents and teens, which can result in the teens feeling less motivated about making any changes. You can discover for yourself, with some guidance in this book, the optimal time to get out of and into bed. If you need to go to bed and get up earlier, you can use techniques to gradually shift toward an earlier time, and you can achieve this by setting realistic goals and moving slowly toward your eventual goal. Behavior change is more successful when it involves wins along the way. Setting an unrealistic goal that is not achievable is frustrating, and since it will be unsuccessful, it can lead to unhelpful self-criticism and equally unhelpful family arguments.

You can also encourage others to read this book, such as your parents, or someone else who works with you, such as a guidance counselor, doctor, or teacher. Reading this book may help them understand how to best support your sleep-related changes.

Too often, the sleep problems of teens are normalized as "just a normal part of teen life," but those problems are in fact treatable, and it is important to treat them to ensure that you do not go on to develop other health-related problems. If you have already developed issues with anxiety, depression, or substance use, this book provides strategies that can help you make changes even while you are struggling with these other problems.

WHY MOST SLEEP ADVICE SEEMS UNHELPFUL

Have you tried to fix your sleep problem, only to find that you don't get the results you want? Have your parents or teachers given you advice that seems impossible to follow? The problem is that teens live in environments that are not suited to their biology, and they are not kids either, so strict schedules and aiming for impossibly high sleep results are unrealistic. Teens experience a shift in their body clock that makes them sleepy later, makes them ready to wake up much later, and makes them more alert later in the day relative to kids and most adults. This shift is temporary and will gradually shift toward something a little earlier during adulthood, but meanwhile we need a book that recognizes this problem and provides real, practical solutions.

Most teens do not suffer only from insomnia; they often also experience daytime sleepiness and excessive sleeping on the weekend. So adult insomnia treatments retrofitted for teens are not helpful and can result in feeling frustrated with the poor results. You need solutions to cope in a world in which your body clock is out of synch with your school hours. You need to be able to wind down and quiet your mind earlier at night. You need practical tips for getting out of bed in the morning. And you also need help feeling more alert during the day. This book is organized around providing tips to solve each of these problems.

This book will provide solutions that use sleep science and con-sider the unique biology and life demands of young adults. Central in these tips is the idea that improvement comes with tracking your sleep, learning about your sleep, coming up with a plan for change, and checking whether you are satisfied with the results of your plan. This book contains state-of-the-art techniques for helping you sleep and feel better. Which tips you select and work on and what goals you set are entirely up to you.

WHO SHOULD USE THIS BOOK?

- Teens who want better sleep and want to feel more alert during the day.

- Parents who want to understand and help with the sleep problems of their teens.

- Those who work with teens and young adults. This includes teachers, professors, guidance counselors, mental health pro-viders, members of family health teams, and pediatricians.

WHO SHOULD NOT USE THIS BOOK?

This book was written specifically for teens with the following sleep problems: not being able to fall asleep quickly; waking up in the middle of the night and not being able to return quickly to sleep; falling asleep during the day; and feeling like you need to sleep for long periods of time on the weekends. The assumption is that these problems are associated with a pubertal shift in the body clock combined with behaviors such as an irregular or ill-timed schedule for getting into and out of bed, an inadequate wind-down period, anxiety or stress, switching between too much or too little time in bed, sleep or alertness-interfering substances or medications, and unhelpful beliefs about sleep.

There are other possible causes for some sleep problems in teens, including sleep disorders such as obstructive sleep apnea or narcolepsy. It is important to have a thorough sleep evaluation or obtain a referral to a sleep specialist to check for alternative explanations for your sleep problems. Although the treatments in this book are suitable for those who also have issues with pain, depression, trauma, or anxiety, these treatments may not be suitable for those with bipolar disorder, seizure disorder, or disorders in which there may be an exacerbation of symptoms when experiencing sleep deprivation. If you have any of these conditions, talk to your doctor. A professional should monitor your treatment, rather than you using a self-management program that could exacerbate your condition.

If you are using mind-altering medications or substances, you may not experience much improvement without decreasing or stopping use of these substances. Some drugs will disrupt the sleep of those with even the most perfect of sleep habits. You may need a doctor's help to stop substance use, and your doctor should be consulted before changing anything related to your medication.

Lastly, if you have significant stress in your life, like grief, homelessness, family conflict, or trauma, consider that it may be unrealistic to expect to sleep well without getting some help for the other issues. There are people who can help you (see the link below), and it may be helpful to get some stability in these areas before beginning a demanding self-management program.

For an extensive list of readings and resources on teen sleep problems and other related issues (crisis hotlines, substance abuse, eating disorders, chronic pain, depression and anxiety, and so on), see the "Suggested Readings and Resources" at http://www.new harbinger.com/44383. That site also includes several downloadable forms for use in connection with this book. See the very back of this book for more details.

A NOTE TO PARENTS AND OTHERS IN THE LIVES OF YOUNG ADULTS

Thank you for reading this book. You understand that sleep problems are not just something that teens need to accept. You understand that there are evidence-based treatments available to them. You may have tried to implement some strategies in the past, and felt frustrated by their ineffectiveness. This is a new approach, one in which young adults can learn about sleep and then set goals they believe they can achieve. Teens need to set their own goals in a way that seems manageable to them, so that they can experience success along the way. Once they have the information, they can make decisions that will ultimately make them feel better, more alert, and more well rested. This is difficult for well-intentioned parents, who may try to push their teen to change sleep habits when the teen is unwilling.

Enforcing a strict schedule, which does not take into account the delay in circadian phase that teens experience, can inadvertently create insomnia. Moreover, teens can develop negative attitudes about regularity, and they may then reject the idea of a regular schedule when they gain control over their schedule (for example, when they go away to college). Likewise, it is more effective to negotiate a shutdown of electronics collaboratively and flexibly than to attempt to take them all away and create a focus on trying to gain access to these devices.

It is supportive to check in and ask if you can help, but it is also helpful for teens to be in charge of their own sleep habits. It is important to be patient with young adults' choices in goal setting. The goal setting may not be exactly what you would want, but it is better to make some movement toward goals than none at all. Lastly, you yourself can model good sleep habits, which includes powering down your own electronic devices and engaging in a regularly timed winddown period in the hour before bed. There are lots of opportunities to positively impact the lives of teens with this simple book, and I applaud you for engaging in this journey with your young adult.

To those who work with teens, this is a book you can use in your work with them. You may have experienced frustration with the help available, both in terms of available treatment providers and in the types of evidence-based treatment material on the market. Because sex hormones create a unique developmental shift in circadian patterns, young adults cannot use children's cognitive behavioral resources. Teens are resistant to the enforcement of unrealistic bedtimes, creating a power struggle and an unhealthy attitude toward schedules. Adult resources are a challenge as well, since some strategies could make things worse. For example, the adult strategy of getting up when you cannot sleep and engaging in an activity until sleepiness returns can result in teens engaging in stimulating activity, staying up a good part of the night, and then having to get up early for school. This normally effective strategy could result in excessive daytime sleepiness and weekend oversleeping. Unlike most adults with insomnia, many teens are not particularly concerned about being awake during the night because of their shifted circadian clock; the bigger complaint is how they feel during the day. They have their own unique sleep problems and few resources to help them.

Existing books for teens focus mainly on getting more hours of sleep. This is only one problem teens face—their sleep problems are far more complex. This book focuses on creating an environment for change rather than inflexibly dictating standards for sleep behaviors that even many adults could not abide. Although sleep duration guidelines are important, rigidly prescribing a schedule of 8.5 hours each night ignores the fact that sleep needs vary: some young adults will require more and some will require less. Allowing teens to discover their current sleep need and then supporting their efforts to engage in behaviors that provide a steady dose of that amount of sleep, or that set the stage for better quality sleep, are much more likely to succeed.

There is considerable misinformation in the media and other sources about sleep, so it is important for you to do your own research when it comes to what advice you give to teens. It is unlikely that teens will follow strict prescriptions to shut down all devices hours before bed, and in any case this may not address the sleep problem. Many books are written solely for parents and don't take into account the teens' perspective. Such books can set up an unhelpful power struggle. Using teens' natural inclination toward self-management, and supporting their work, can allow them to achieve their own goals and feel efficacious about their sleep health habits. Books like this one, or my free companion self-management app DOZe (also sometimes referred to as *doze*), can be recommended to teens, with an offer to check in on results and provide support along the way. I invite you to read this book and provide a cheerleading role as teens make healthy sleep choices. Teens will ask for help when they need it. Waiting for an invitation to the process can make you a powerful ally. Thank you for reading this book and for all that you do to help make young adults' lives better.

Summary

- Sleep problems are highly prevalent in young adults.

- There are evidence-based tools available, but many have not been adapted to the unique problems of young adults, or it may be difficult to access appropriate tools.

- Young adults like to make their own decisions and set their own goals—they like to self-manage.

- This book is organized around evidence-based tips to improve sleep. In each tip chapter, learning about sleep, tracking your own sleep, and goal setting are the keys to improvement. You are encouraged to (1) identify and understand the problem; (2) come up with a solution, choosing from solutions proven to work; (3) set a goal; and (4) check if you are pleased with the result.

Identify Your Sleep Problem with the Right Tool: The Sleep Tracker

If there is one thing I talk about to people with sleep problems more than anything else, it's that in order to change a problem, you have to understand the problem. If you want to understand your sleep, then you need to observe your sleep.

"But I already know what my sleep is like..." It's possible that you are an exception to the rule, but many studies have shown that people tend to remember their habits as more regular than they are.

Here is an example. Brett is a freshman in high school and he told me that he always goes to bed by 10 p.m. and always gets up by 6:30 a.m. and that it always takes him about two hours to fall asleep. Brett completed a Sleep Tracker monitoring form for me. (Brett's Sleep Tracker can be viewed and downloaded at http://www.new harbinger.com/44383.) He found that over the course of two weeks he went to bed later than 10 p.m. on 80% of the nights. There was also about four hours of variability in the time at which he went to bed, because there were a few weekend nights in which he went to bed later than 2 a.m. Although his alarm was set for 6:45 a.m., Brett rarely got out of bed at that time; in contrast to weekend mornings, on weekends he occasionally got out of bed as late as 1:30 p.m. That is, there was a variability or difference of about seven hours between the earliest and latest rise times. There were four nights in which it took him close to two hours to fall asleep, but there were several nights in which he fell asleep very quickly (within about five minutes), and on most nights he fell asleep within a normal amount of time (namely, in under thirty minutes).

So why wasn't Brett accurate about his sleep patterns? People tend to remember things that are consistent with their overall perception of the problem. If you have a problem falling asleep, for example, you may focus on the worst few nights of falling asleep and you may unintentionally forget about the few good nights. If I asked you right now to answer a few questions about your sleep last week or even last night, you probably would not be very accurate. But if tomorrow morning, as soon as you woke up, you were to answer the same questions, your answers would be much more accurate.

SHOULD WE MEASURE SLEEP BY MEASURING BRAIN WAVE ACTIVITY?

There are a lot of misconceptions about what sleep is and how we can measure it. You may be aware that during an overnight sleep study, patients wear electrodes all over their head to measure brain activity. Sleep is considered to be "sleep" when we see a particular brain wave activity on the EEG (electroencephalograph) for a certain amount of time. But there is a potential problem with this definition. Here is what happens as you fall asleep: your brain waves slow and are characterized by electrical activity we call theta. Your eyes often start to roll back into their sockets, producing slow eye-rolling movements. Your muscle tone starts to decrease as you relax. You are thought to be "asleep" when over half of the 30-second period we are examining on the EEG is characterized by sleep brain waves. However, this means that if for 14 seconds of a 30-second period you were awake, but there were 16 seconds in which you were in the lightest stage of sleep, this is called "sleep." This is probably why many people, when woken from this stage of sleep, say they were not sleeping at all. So this way we measure and define sleep (that is, as electrical activity) misses the experience of sleepers. So if electrical activity does not provide a perfect way of capturing sleep, what else is there?

SHOULD WE MEASURE SLEEP BY MEASURING PHYSICAL ACTIVITY?

There are many devices or apps you can buy (fitness trackers, for example) that supposedly measure sleep. These tools do not directly measure sleep but assume there are certain physical movements you make during sleep that are not typical of when you are awake, and vice versa. Is it true that these devices can tell you whether you are asleep just by your movements? Not really. What if you are a very restless sleeper or a sleeper who moves very little? The devices may be okay for getting an overall sense of when people are awake and at rest, but sleep doctors do not use them because the estimates are not accurate enough, and also because they are linked to users becoming more preoccupied with sleep, anxiety, and insomnia. That is, people who use them tend to become overly obsessed with "biohacking" and measuring aspects of themselves, even when the measurements are inaccurate, and this makes them feel more anxious about sleep.

WHY SLEEP TRACKERS ARE THE BEST TOOL FOR HELPING WITH INSOMNIA

So what is a Sleep Tracker? It is a monitoring form in which you track your sleep behaviors and your experiences. Just as you might monitor the food you eat if you want to make eating changes, monitoring what you experience as sleep will help you make changes to your sleep habits. You can download the Sleep Tracker daily form and weekly form at http://www.newharbinger.com/44383.

Insomnia is a disorder in which people are complaining about the experience of not being able to sleep well. So it is important to get an understanding of your experience as well as your habits. Most of the items that are on a Sleep Tracker are items that require no estimations and are relatively easy, like when you got into bed last night or the last time you woke you up. Other items focus on your experience as a sleeper. An example of an item that asks for your experience is, "How long did it feel like it took you to fall asleep?" This question is a little harder to answer objectively for the reasons we discussed above, so it should be a guesstimate based on your experience. If it felt like it took two hours, write that down. Once your sleep starts to improve, you may estimate this as far less than two hours, so we don't fret over whether this is 100% accurate. Indeed, watching the clock to try to provide a more "objectively precise" estimate of the time it took to fall asleep would make your sleep and anxiety worse. A guesstimate is better.

WHAT IF YOU "DON'T SLEEP"?

When people fail to perceive the moment they fall asleep, they may conclude that they "didn't sleep a wink." But even when people experience what they believe to be "no sleep at all," night after night, they continue to lay in bed with their eyes closed and the lights off for normal amounts of time (for example, eight hours). That is, they do not shorten their time in bed and engage in other activities, to take advantage of their new found apparent lack of need for sleep. They continue to go to bed at the same time and spend hours lying there, experiencing it as wakefulness. When asked to talk about what happened during the eight hours of time in bed awake, they are unable to provide many details other than, "I lay there, resting my eyes, for eight hours." Their daytime impairment is typically no different from people who sleep much more.

Sound familiar? If you have this kind of insomnia, are awake at 11:43 p.m., and look at the clock at 2:32 a.m., you might simply assume the time between 11:43 and 2:32 was wakefulness. Fortunately, even if you feel like you "don't sleep," you are still able to benefit from the strategies in this book. Remind yourself that it is not possible to "not sleep" for anything more than a day or so.

Continue to use the Sleep Tracker, but know that once you start to follow the advice, you are likely to see big improvements that will be in part due to your returned ability to detect when you fall sleep (in addition to sleep improvements).

USE THE ONE, TWO, THREE PLAN

If you are unhappy with your sleep, use the Sleep Tracker to help you get better sleep in three easy steps.

1. First, complete the Sleep Tracker for two weeks. It's simple: Answer eight questions each day to get to know your sleep habits and sleep characteristics. Using the downloadable Weekly Sleep Tracker or the DOZe app might be most helpful.

2. Second, learn how to improve your sleep by reading this book. Make a sleep plan.

3. Third, try your sleep plan for two weeks while completing the Sleep Tracker. At the end of the two weeks you can see how your sleep has improved, and either stop, maintain the same plan, or add or replace goals and track for two more weeks.

THE SLEEP TRACKER QUESTIONS

Each morning for two weeks, as soon as you get up, complete these eight easy questions:

1. About what time did you get into bed? (This time may be different from when you actually turned off the light and tried to fall asleep.)

2. About what time did you turn off the light and try to fall asleep? (Record the time that you began trying to fall asleep.)

3. How long did it take you to fall asleep? (Record how long you guess it took you to fall asleep. We know this can be hard to guess since you probably didn't look at the clock just before you feel asleep! Just give your best estimate.)

4. If you woke up during your sleep, how long were you awake in total? (What do you record if you woke up more than once in the night? If you think you woke up three times for about 20 minutes each, record 1 hour. This should be your best guess; it doesn't need to be exact.)

5. When did you finally wake up in the morning? (A good way to define this is: At what time did your body last wake up for the day—whether it was because of an alarm, a parent or roommate waking you up, or any other reason. Record the time you woke up, not the time you got out of bed.)

6. What time did you get out of bed for the day? (Record the time you got out of bed and didn't try to go back to sleep.)

7. How long did you nap or doze yesterday? (A nap is when you decided to sleep during the day. Dozing is a time you nodded off without meaning to, for example, while watching TV.)

8. Did you eat, drink, or smoke any sleep-interfering products yesterday? (For example, cigarettes, alcohol, marijuana, narcotics, coffee, tea, or an energy drink. You may wonder why we are lumping behaviors like narcotic use with something as seemingly benign as tea. Many teens are concerned that their parents could see that they use marijuana or cigarettes, so to encourage monitoring, we keep it general. This way, you can keep track and feel comfortable that this disclosure won't get you into trouble.)

HINTS FOR COMPLETING THE SLEEP TRACKER

When you are writing down details about your sleep, the closer you are to when you woke up, the more accurate it will be, so try to prioritize completing it early in the morning. You may find that leaving the Sleep Tracker questions with a pen (if it is on paper) on your nightstand or desk, or, if it is on your computer, leaving it at the breakfast table, may increase the likelihood that you will do it consistently and accurately.

There is also a free Sleep Tracker app for young adults called DOZe, developed by the author of this book, downloadable at www .dozeapp.ca. DOZe is a self-management tool that allows you to track your sleep on your phone, receive feedback about your sleep, access information about how to sleep well, and set goals for sleeping better. Its tracking feature can be used instead of the paper Sleep Tracker.

What to Do with the Sleep Tracker Information

There are many important things you can learn from your Sleep Tracker. It can tell you about your sleep patterns over time, as well as about behaviors that may get in the way of sleeping well or feeling alert during the day. Let's go through some of the things you may want to know about your sleep. First, a summary of how you are sleeping.

1. Falling asleep: This estimate of how long it took you to fall asleep is taken directly from item 3 of the Sleep Tracker (see above). You can calculate an average by adding this value from each night during the two weeks you collected the information and then divide by the number of days you monitored. Apps like DOZe automatically make this calculation, and all the calculations below, for you. Generally speaking, it should take somewhere between ten to thirty minutes to fall asleep. If your average is within this range, but you have one or perhaps two nights in which you take longer than thirty minutes, this is considered normal. Taking more than thirty minutes to fall asleep on average is suggestive of insomnia. Taking less than ten minutes to fall asleep suggests that there is a problem with sleepiness.

2. Staying asleep: This is taken from item 4 of the Sleep Tracker. Generally speaking, you should be awake less than thirty minutes during the night. If your average is above this amount, it suggests that you have insomnia. If your average is within this range, but you have one or perhaps two nights

in which you are awake longer than thirty minutes, this is considered normal.

3. Time spent in bed: This is calculated from the difference between the time you got into bed (item 1) and the time at which you got out of bed (item 6). If your average time in bed is between 8 and 10.5 hours (if you are 14–17 years old) or 7–9 hours (if you are 18–25 years old), this is probably a healthy amount of time. If it is less than 8 hours (if you are 14–17 years old) or less than 7 hours (if you are 18–25 years old), this is probably too short. If it is above 10.5 hours for those 14–17 years old, or above 9.5 hours for those 18–25 years old, this is probably too much time in bed.

4. Total sleep time: Another important index is how much time you are sleeping. You can determine your total sleep time by subtracting any time that you are awake in bed from your sleep opportunity, in other words, the amount of time that you were in bed for the purposes of sleep (the number calculated in #3 above). Wakeful time in bed includes: (1) the time it took for you to fall asleep, (2) the time you spent awake in the middle of the night, and (3) the time that was spent awake in bed in the morning before getting out of bed (the difference between Sleep Tracker items 5 and 6). If you are 14–17 years old and you sleep an average of 8–10 hours, or you are 18–25 years old and sleep an average of 7–9 hours, this is considered healthy. Your average sleep time may be too short if it is less than 7 hours

(if you are 14–17 years old) or less than 6 hours (if you are 18–25 years old). Your average sleep length may be too long if it is over 10 hours (if you are 14–17 years old) or over 9 hours (if you are 18–25 years old).

HOW TO BECOME UNSTUCK ABOUT USING THE SLEEP TRACKER

If you have trouble getting started with the Sleep Tracker because you worry that it will make your sleep worse or that you won't get it perfect, you should know that sleep tends to improve, albeit not to a large degree, just by monitoring. Think about eating. Most people who want to make a change in their eating habits don't like the idea of monitoring, but monitoring eating sheds light on places to change (for example, high-calorie snacks or eating late at night). A Sleep Tracker is no different. It tells you which areas need to change, it allows you to make a plan, and it tracks whether the plan has resulted in improvement. Tracking your sleep will not make your sleep worse.

Similarly, if you are concerned that you cannot track your sleep "perfectly," most people realize that it is not necessary or even desirable to approach the Sleep Tracker with perfection as a goal. However, if you remain anxious about using the Tracker, even after this reassurance that it will not make your sleep worse and does not have to be done "perfectly," we recommend that you skip ahead to Tip 9: "Think Like a Good Sleeper." After completing the Tip 9 chapter, you may be able to engage with the other Tips in this book, which require the use of the Sleep Tracker.

Summary

- Knowledge is power. Tracking your sleep every morning is the best way to learn about your sleep and sleep patterns.

- Devices are based on assumptions about the nature of sleep (for example, that sleep is about movement, brain activity, or heart rate), but when it comes to insomnia, they don't give you what you want: information about your behavior and your experience of sleeplessness.

- Use the One, Two, Three plan. Step One is to track your sleep for two weeks with the Sleep Tracker. Step Two is to read a Tip chapter and make a plan for change. Step Three is to try out your new sleep plan and track your sleep for two weeks to determine if you are getting the sleep results that you wanted. You can use the free DOZe app if it would help to track it on your phone with reminders.

Your Plan for the Week

Determine your plan for the week:

☐ Find a place for my Sleep Tracker (next to my bed or at the breakfast table), or download the DOZe app to make it more likely for me to remember.

☐ Set a notification on my phone to remind me to complete the Sleep Tracker (DOZe will email you each morning).

☐ Track sleep every morning within an hour of waking up.

☐ I don't feel ready to track my sleep. I will skip to Tip 9 to examine my beliefs about my sleep. (All the other Tips rely on sleep information provided by the Tracker.)

Use Your Body Clock to Get Better Sleep and Feel Better During the Day

Did you know that if you are having sleeping problems and feel tired, moody, or mentally foggy, it could be due to a hidden problem with your body clock? You may have noticed that your body clock has shifted later than it was when you were a child, so that you feel alert later into the night and feel unable to get out of bed early in the morning. This late-shifted body rhythm can place you at odds with the demands in your life. You may even become so tired from the lack of sleep that you try to make up for it by oversleeping on the weekends or hitting the snooze button on your alarm and skipping breakfast because you don't yet feel ready to get up.

The result of this scenario is that the timing of when you do things, such as getting into and out of bed, going outside for the first time in the day, and eating meals, can become very irregular. Your body clock is desperately looking for regularity, but what it gets is a jumbled, ever-shifting mess. An ever-shifting body clock can make you feel tired and unable to sleep when you want and wake up when you want.

If this sounds familiar, don't worry. There is a solution, and it starts with understanding your body clock and how to use it to achieve your sleep and alertness goals. In this chapter, you will learn that a jumbled schedule results in symptoms that are the same as jet lag, without having traveled: symptoms like fatigue, concentration difficulties, and feeling moody. Later in the chapter you can use your Sleep Tracker to spot those "jet lag without travel" symptoms.

WHAT IS A BODY CLOCK?

Your body actually contains many clocks, and the brain coordinates all of them. These clocks control many things, including hormones, sleepiness, alertness, mood, body temperature, eating, and your optimal sleep window. If you graphed any of your body clocks' activity, you would see a curved line that rises and falls in a predictable way every day. For example, the central body clock in the brain controls alertness, which typically rises and falls reliably over a 24-hour period. You would see very little alerting signal from the brain in the morning hours (sound familiar?), but in the afternoon you would see increasing alertness until it reaches a peak in the evening, and then your alertness signal falls at night.

Does this explain how you feel during the day? Do you feel not at all alert in the early morning and not start to feel very alert until the afternoon? Do you feel at your mental best in the late afternoon and evening? Is it difficult to wind down at night to go to bed until very late? Whatever your pattern, this is your body clock and its alerting signal at work, and this chapter will teach you how to set your body clock so that it works for you and your schedule.

Give Your Body Clock Regular Clues to Tell It What Time It Is

Your body clock system pays very careful attention to cues in the environment to tell it what time it is. Environmental cues include sunlight, food, movement, and going to bed, but also chemicals in your brain, like melatonin, a hormone regularly released in the evening that signals that sleep will occur later that night. If you live where Daylight Savings is observed, you will notice that during this one-hour shift, your body takes note of the discrepancy between the time of the clock and the shift. The clock is aware that the sun is not in the expected place in the sky (that is, it is either lighter or darker than expected), even though this is only a one-hour difference. Because the internal clock is set by cues in the environment and behaviors, consistency in your daily schedule will help your clock run efficiently.

Light: Neither Friend nor Foe of the Clock

Behaviors such as bedtime and eating help set our body's clock, but you've probably also noticed quite a lot of talk about light and smartphones as things that influence your internal clock as well. Your brain has many connections to the eye. Before we had artificial light, your body clock relied on seeing the sun rising and setting and the absence of light at night to tell it what time it was. Now that we could have 24 hours of darkness or light by controlling a light switch, there are plenty of opportunities for your clock to get confused.

You may remember from science class that you see colors in a visible spectrum, including blue and violet at one pole. The sun produces blue light, and blue light is important for setting the clock and making you feel alert. Ideally, you would have lots of sunlight in the morning and throughout the day to help you feel alert. Bright light should fade somewhat in the evening hours, as this is when the sun sets. Many of your electronic devices emit blue light, as do LED (light-emitting diode) bulbs. This is why it has been argued that there should be an absence of blue light sources in the evening, because blue light in the hours before bed can trick the clock into thinking it is earlier than it is. But remember, blue light is an important part of the day that helps with daytime alertness and sets the stage for healthy sleep at night. If you don't have much daylight available to you, you can use artificial lights to try and send a message to your clock. Getting plenty of daylight might also mean going for a walk in the sunlight during spare-time or lunch periods at school, or walking home from school at the end of the day.

Why Do You Need an Efficient, Regulated Clock?

If your clock controls sleep, alertness, mood, and hormones, a clock that runs well allows you to sleep when needed, wake when needed, feel physically and mentally alert when needed, and remain in a positive or neutral mood. In other words, your clock works with your goals, not against them. Think about what adults do for little kids when it comes to regulating their clocks. They put them to bed around the same time, they feed them around the same time, they wake them up around the same time—kids have routines and adults tend to be protective of those routines. What if you invited someone over with small children for a dinner at 8 p.m.—how do you think the parent would react? How would the children react? We would expect that the children's mood would be cranky because they may be up later and eating later than their clock is used to. Although we unfortunately tend to forget this fact, even as adults we remain clock creatures and we need regular input into the clock for the clock-related systems to work best.

HOW DO YOU KNOW IF YOU HAVE A WELL-REGULATED CLOCK?

A well-regulated body clock means that you get sleepy and fall asleep around the same time each night and wake up spontaneously and consistently around the same time in the morning. You have an optimal "window" of time, specific to you, in which you are most likely to sleep well. When you sleep in synch with this window, you fall asleep within a normal amount of time (about 10–30 minutes) and are able to wake up without too much difficulty. If your body clock receives regular cues (that is, you go to bed and get up around the same time each day and have regular light exposure), you will feel relatively alert throughout the day. You will also feel hungry around the same times during the day, and in general your mood will remain fairly neutral or positive. If this does not sound like your experience currently, don't worry—making some changes will make you feel better.

SUFFERING FROM "JET LAG SYMPTOMS WITHOUT EVEN TRAVELING"?

Jet lag is a helpful way to understand how your internal clock affects sleep, and how you feel during the day. Jet lag occurs when there is a mismatch between the internal body clock and the environment, and it results in symptoms such as fatigue, mood changes, upset stomach, mental fogginess, and wanting to sleep or eat or be awake at odd times.

Jet lag can occur in two different scenarios:

1. *Travel across time zones:* If you were to fly to London, England, which is six hours ahead of New York time, your body would remain on New York time for the first little part of your trip until your body readjusted, over the course of a day or two, to the new time through exposure to light and dark and meals on London time.

2. *An irregular schedule (especially an irregular wake-up time):* When you have an irregular schedule, the same mismatch between the internal body clock and the environment occurs. For example, if you wake up at 7 a.m. on weekdays and then 12 noon on weekends, your body clock gets "reset" on weekends by the new wake-up time of 12 noon. Your body clock shifts forward by five hours, meaning that you will likely have more difficulty falling asleep at your bedtime on Sunday night and you will likely experience symptoms of jet lag when you have to reset your clock on Monday morning at the beginning of the school week. This is the physical equivalent of flying to Hawaii and back over the

course of the weekend. And it may be every weekend for some teens.

Use Your Sleep Tracker to Find Jet Lag, and Get Rid of It

Take a moment to look at your sleep-tracking data, ideally over the past two weeks. Examine the difference in hours (that is, the number of time zones you crossed without actually traveling) between the earliest and latest times at which you:

1. Went to bed (item 1).

2. Attempted to go to sleep (item 2).

3. Woke up for the last time (item 5).

4. Got out of bed (item 6).

Alternatively, you can use the free DOZe app, and it will provide a "jet lag without travel" index for you. The DOZe app will also help you with your goals in this chapter. Each hour is equivalent to a time zone—the greater the number of time zones, the greater the severity of the jet lag symptoms and the longer it will take to adjust physically. For example, if your earliest bedtime was 10 p.m. and the latest was 1:30 a.m., this creates over 3 hours of difference, which is equivalent, physiologically speaking, to flying from Los Angeles to New York City. If you are traveling a time zone or more on any of these indices, you may find yourself experiencing jet lag symptoms.

We blame how terrible we feel on Monday, but many of us essentially take a trip without ever traveling from Sunday to Monday most weeks. To get rid of or minimize jet lag, you want to manage the variability. There are life demands, including early-morning extracurricular activities or going out with friends at night, that may interfere with maintaining a steady bedtime and rise time every single day, but creating a regular schedule with occasional changes to go with the flow of life demands will make a big difference in the way you feel during the day and how you sleep at night.

SET A GOAL TO MANAGE "JET LAG WITHOUT TRAVEL"

You may wonder how much variability is okay; that is, to avoid the symptoms of jet lag, does your schedule need to have zero variability? Probably not. You probably value some spontaneity and you should sleep to live, not live to sleep, so prioritizing a completely rigid schedule over all other activities is not a balanced way of approaching regulating your clock. That said, your body craves regular input into its clock system, and you want to get as close to that as possible without sacrificing the reasons you want to get good sleep in the first place. A rule of thumb is that one hour of variability is mild, but perceivable. Reducing your variability down to an hour or less is best, though that may not be a realistic goal for everyone.

If you are currently suffering from concentration, fatigue, sleep, or mood problems, why not set a goal for two weeks that reduces the variability and track your results? If you met your goal but you are still dissatisfied with how you feel, consider cutting out another hour of variability.

UNDERSTANDING HOW YOUR CLOCK CHANGES AS YOU GET OLDER

You've learned about the important role of behavior, that is, keeping variability for "into bed" and "out of bed" times to a minimum, but there are also other factors that affect the clock. There are both developmental and genetic components to your body clock system.

Your clock changes with different life stages. Young children tend to have early bedtimes and rise times, which means that they tend to get sleepy early, get hungry early, and wake up early. You have probably noticed that little kids tend to be rather extreme early birds. With the onset of puberty, bedtimes, rise times, and mealtimes tend to shift backward so you get sleepy later, have difficulty waking up early, and delay when you first eat. Many teens become extreme night owls and will remain this way until they are through puberty, and often until they begin a job that requires them to get up earlier five days per week. Teens tend to increase their lateness by engaging in activities later and later, which makes the shift toward lateness more pronounced, but even without these behaviors, teens have a developmental preference for lateness. You will likely spend most of your adulthood somewhere in between a night owl and an early bird's schedule until later adulthood, when, once again, we see a developmental shift toward being an early bird. This is why we see senior citizens eating dinner very early, falling asleep early in the evening, and waking up very early in the morning.

Your clock is genetically determined. In addition to the developmental component of your clock, there is a genetic component that determines your "chronotype," that is, whether you are a morning person or a night owl, or whether you are somewhere in between. For example, if you have always been a night owl since early childhood, you probably have a biological parent who is, and always has been, a night owl. Parents who are night owls often have to get up early to take care of their children, so it may not be obvious that one of your parents is a night owl.

Why does it matter that your body clock type, or as we call it, your "chronotype," is genetic? It matters because that means it is somewhat difficult to alter drastically. If you have always been a night owl, you are unlikely to shift into being an early bird. Does this mean you can't shift your rhythm at all? Not exactly. You will learn below that your clock is always looking for steady cues, so if you provide regular cues to the clock that are consistent with an earlier rhythm, it will be easier for you to get sleepy earlier and get up earlier.

SELF-TEST: ARE YOU LIVING AS A NIGHT OWL IN AN EARLY BIRD'S WORLD?

Answer these questions to see if your body clock is shifted relative to other people's.

1. What time would you get out of bed if you paid attention only to when you feel your physical best?

    (0) If it is before 8 a.m., this is fairly typical of an early bird.

    (1) If it is 8–10 a.m., this is somewhere in between an early bird and a night owl.

    (2) If it is after 10 a.m., you are likely a night owl.

2. What time would you get into bed for the purposes of sleep (that is, not watching television or other wakeful activities) if you paid attention only to when you are feeling sleepy?

    (0) If it is before 10 p.m., this is fairly typical of an early bird.

    (1) If it is between 10 p.m. and midnight, this is somewhere in between an early bird and a night owl.

    (2) If it is after midnight, this is most consistent with a night owl.

3. Generally speaking, how easy is it for you to get out of bed in the morning?

    (0) If it is very easy, this is fairly typical of an early bird.

    (1) If it is only somewhat difficult, this is somewhere in between an early bird and a night owl.

    (2) If it is very difficult, this is most typical of a night owl.

4. At what time in the evening do you feel sleepy and in need of sleep?

    (0) If it is before 10 p.m., this is fairly typical of an early bird.

    (1) If it is between 10 p.m. and midnight, this is somewhere in between an early bird and a night owl.

    (2) If it is after midnight, this is most consistent with a night owl.

5. If you could schedule your examinations for school based on when you would feel most alert, which of the times below would you pick?

(0) If it is before 10 a.m., this is fairly typical of an early bird.

(1) If it is between 11 a.m. and 3 p.m., this is somewhere in between an early bird and a night owl.

(2) If it is after 5 p.m., this is most consistent with a night owl.

Results (add up your above responses):

0–3: Early bird

4–6: Flexible; neither an early bird nor a night owl

7–10: Night owl

Tips for early birds: Those with scores typical of an early bird are shifted earlier than most people. This means that as long as you prioritize winding down an hour before bed, you should be able to have an early enough bedtime (say, 10 p.m.) to get enough sleep.

- Prioritize winding down about an hour before bed and go to bed when you feel sleepy.

- Keep your schedule regular.

- Do not sleep in on weekends more than *one hour* later than your weekday rise time.

Tips for those who are flexible (that is, neither early birds nor night owls): Your weekday wake-up schedule may be slightly earlier than suits you biologically, but you are flexible to minor shifts (of about an hour or so), and your schedule is probably not too far off your optimal schedule. Many teens will eventually become flexible chronotypes as adults unless they were night owls prior to puberty (that is, when they were children).

- Prioritize winding down at least an hour before bed in order to get to bed early enough (say, 10 p.m.) to get enough sleep.

- Set your alarm for as late as possible so that you can get as much sleep as you can. It may help if you move some of your morning routine (such as showering, choosing your clothes, and making your lunch) to the evening before.

- Keep your schedule regular and get lots of light exposure and movement as soon as you wake up in the morning and throughout the daylight hours.

- Limit sleeping in on weekends to no later than 9 a.m.

Tips for night owls: If you are a night owl, some behaviors can shift your circadian rhythm even later. For example, if you do activities later, especially with active engagement under well-lighted conditions, and if you sleep in whenever possible, it will make your night owl tendency even more pronounced. This is why it is important to decrease blue light exposure and exposure to alerting activities early in the evening. If you need to wake up on school days at 7 a.m. or earlier, you will need to engage in a set of habits that help you shift your clock a little earlier, to help you fall asleep earlier and make it physiologically easier to get up earlier too. This will require you to stay on this schedule on the weekends too, or all your hard work during the week will be quickly undone on the weekend. Here are some tips:

- Prioritize winding down two hours before bed in order to get to bed early to get enough sleep. This will mean switching to modes on devices that eliminate blue light and disengaging from activities that make you feel more alert (such as gaming or engaging in socially charged activities like phone calls or social media). Switch to more passive forms of winding down like reading, television, or other hobbies. If this continues to be a problem, please read the chapters for Tips 3 and 4.

- Keep your schedule regular, with a focus on getting as much light exposure as possible as soon as possible after waking up. (Sunlight is the most ideal source of this light, so try going for a walk.) Getting up at a regular time and setting your body clock with light and movement will gradually shift your clock earlier, making it easier to wake up early on following mornings. Do not wear hoodies or keep blinds closed and lights off as you walk around the house first thing in the morning.

- On weekends, try not to sleep more than 1–2 hours later than your regular weekday wake-up time. Every hour you spend sleeping in on weekend mornings makes weekday mornings feel even worse, because you are keeping your clock shifted late; it also makes it that much harder to fall asleep during the week.

- Increasing the regularity of your daytime activities (exposure to light first thing in the morning, early wind-down bedtime routine, three meals taken around 7 a.m., 12 noon, and 6 p.m.) also helps your body clock set itself on a regular schedule.

Summary

- Your internal clock determines when you are most likely to be wakeful, sleepy, hungry, and so on, so you have an optimum window in which your body is more likely to produce the best quality of sleep.

- The clock is set by environmental events like a morning wake-up time and morning light exposure.

- If you wake up at different times each day, you may produce symptoms of jet lag, as your body clock is "reset" every day.

- Exposing yourself to lots of light during the evening (from computers, tablets, and smartphone screens) can delay your rhythm so that you get sleepy later and have trouble waking up early.

- Along with observing your sleep with the Sleep Tracker, you can track your alertness in the morning, afternoon, and evening. Then, next week, set some goals (using the next chapter) to regulate your clock and write them down. While working on your goals, track your sleep with the Sleep Tracker again, as well as re-rating your alertness in the morning, afternoon, and evening. You can use the Tracking Improvement for Body Clock Changes and Post-Experiment Reflection forms (downloadable at www.new harbinger.com/44383) to help you track progress. You can also use the sleep app DOZe to track your jet lag goals.

Your Plan for the Week

☐ Make a plan to manage "jet lag without travel" by limiting the variability of when you get into bed to sleep and when you get out of bed in the morning to less than one hour.

☐ Assess the effects of decreasing your variability using the Sleep Tracker or the DOZe app.

☐ If you were able to achieve the goal you set above but are still unhappy with the results, consider reducing your variability by at least 30 minutes.

Wind Down Before Bed

Do you stay busy and engaged right up until the time you want to sleep, and then find yourself feeling wide awake in bed? This is one of the most common sleep complaints, and there are solutions to this problem throughout the book, but in this chapter we will focus on a deceptively simple solution: taking an hour or two before bed to prepare for sleep. In other words, establishing an effective wind-down routine.

WHAT IS A WIND-DOWN ROUTINE?

Think back to when you were a kid. What was your wind-down routine before bed? A typical routine is one in which you stop an activity by a certain time, take a bath, get on your pajamas, brush your teeth and hair, and then read with a parent. Even before this pre-bed routine, the "activity" that is stopped before starting the bedtime routine is typically an activity that allows for an easy enough transition to the bedtime routine. Have you ever heard an adult say something like, "You are *never* going to be able to calm down to go to bed," in response to activities like wrestling, watching an emotionally charged program, or playing an exciting video game? When adults complain about certain activities right before bed, it is because they realize that it takes some time to calm down and prepare for sleep both physically and emotionally. The need for disengagement from exciting or activating activities does not go away as you age. If you stay mentally, physically, or emotionally active up until the time you go to bed, you will likely find yourself awake in bed. So a wind-down routine should involve activities that have a low level of excitement or alertness before bed to set the stage for a natural transition to sleep.

WIND DOWN EVERY NIGHT

Every night you need to make a transition from being busy and engaged to a more calm state. Your mind and body need to know that it is time for a new state: a state that is one step closer to your sleep state. By establishing this as a regular habit, you can cue your body into switching into this state with routine. But how do you do this?

Switch Out of Your "Doing" Self and into Your "Being" Self

Mindfulness is a practice in which you pay attention to the present moment, without judgment. It is a state that is helpful for sleep because a mindful state is about just "being." What does this mean? Your "self" during the day is concerned with action, problem-solving, and getting things done. It's an important part of yourself, but it is a self that is not compatible with sleep. Why? To "do" things requires great mental energy and sometimes physical energy, too.

Mental energy is needed to do things because getting things done requires creating a plan and future-oriented thinking to monitor for possible barriers to the plan. This is not compatible with sleep. Your "being" self is not action-oriented and not future-focused. Your being self lives in the present moment, a moment that just is. The being self does not evaluate the present moment as good or bad; it just notices it. Your being self doesn't need to "do" anything; you are valuable and perfect in that particular moment. The being self does not try to change your thoughts or emotions, and it does not try to avoid experiences—the being self simply notices and accepts.

Sleep is not something you "do." Sleep is a process that unfolds naturally and you cannot resist it—sleep will always find a way to happen. If you stay in your daily active mind-set (that is, your doing self) right up until the time you go to bed, you will likely find yourself awake in bed because there is no transition to just being. In thinking about the transition to this self (that is, to the being self), we also need to think about what activities are compatible with this self and whether there are any barriers in the environment that could interfere with this transition.

Minimize Blue Light During Your Wind-Down

As noted in the Tip 2 chapter, blue light is important for sleep because we need it during the day to help with our body clock. But blue light is also alerting, and exposure to it in the early evening can delay the release of melatonin, thereby delaying sleep later in the night. There are ways to minimize blue light exposure from your devices (for example, using the "Night Shift" feature on Apple products, or the f.lux program for your computer), but there may still be some residual blue light exposure with these features. One way to further manage the sleep-delaying properties of blue light is to avoid using devices in close proximity to your face (phones, tablets, and computers) in the hour or two before bed. You can replace these high blue light device activities with lesser blue light activities such as listening to music or podcasts, or watching television. And of course, there are lots of other good wind-down activities that do not involve devices at all (for example, reading without a device), and this would be an ideal option in the hour or so before you intend to go to bed. Challenge your family or roommates to also put away their devices at a certain time. You don't necessarily need to eliminate devices altogether, but the earlier you power down, the better sleep results you will likely get.

Avoid Activities That Leave You Feeling Charged Up

Of course, blue light is not the only alerting factor with devices. Another factor to consider is whether an activity is emotionally alerting or difficult to stop. Gaming is a good example of an activity that can leave you feeling very alert and that may entice you to play long after you intended to stop (see the example of Hamdy, below). There are probably lots of individual differences, and it may depend on what type of game it is. Active gaming (for example, your vantage point is behind the gun your avatar is holding) and violent gaming are more disruptive than more passive, nonviolent games. Violent gaming right before bed produces effects on your physiology even after you fall asleep, so it is a habit that is important to change (you should move this activity much earlier in the evening, or consider stopping altogether if you have disrupted sleep). If you find yourself feeling emotionally activated by an activity you do before bed (see the example of Avida, below, and how group chats left her feeling activated), it is important to experiment with the timing of the disruptive habit, or replace it with something more helpful.

Experiment with Activities

Some young adults do not know what else to do with their time during the wind-down period. If you are unsure of what to do initially, brainstorm ideas ahead of time and write them down. Create a long list of possibilities for your pre-bedtime routine. For example:

- Reading
- Podcasts or audiobooks
- Adult coloring books
- Painting or sketching
- Crafting
- Building models or robotics
- Taking the dog for a walk
- Board games
- Solitaire
- Taking a bath
- Yoga or meditation

What other activities can you think of?

TEST IF YOUR WIND-DOWN ROUTINE WORKS WELL

The answer to whether your wind-down works can be found in the results it produces—that is, are you able to fall asleep within a half an hour of when you intend to sleep? You can double-check this by looking at your sleep information on the Sleep Tracker, or use a free sleep tracking app like DOZe, and look at the average time to fall asleep. We emphasize checking this objectively from a sleep diary because many people assume they have a good wind-down routine, but when they see the tracked result, they are surprised to learn that their routine is not effective. If you do not feel like you are in a sleep-compatible state after your wind-down routine and your Tracker shows that you are not falling asleep within a normal amount of time (that is, under 30 minutes), it may be time to look more critically at your routine.

"I HAVE A WIND-DOWN ROUTINE— IT DOESN'T WORK!"

What if you have a routine that you use to wind down, but you still do not feel like you are prepared for sleep, or it takes you more than 30 minutes to fall asleep? Consider the following cases:

> *Avida does homework until about 9:30 or 10:00 most nights and then wants to wind down after all that work. She picks up her phone to relax and catch up with her friends. She sees her friends are already engaged in a group chat, talking about a fight at school. Avida jumps into the chat and before she knows it, she*

is already an hour past the time at which she should go to bed and she still doesn't want to exit the chat. By the time she decides to go to bed, the most amount of sleep she could possibly get is five hours. Avida feels frustrated thinking about how hard it will be to stay awake in class tomorrow.

Hamdy spends his evenings gaming. He is known as the best of his friends at a particular game and loves playing. Once his friends start dropping out of the online game, Hamdy brings his laptop to bed so that he can play a few more games for practice before going to sleep. After he is finished playing, he sets his laptop on his bedside table, turns out the light, and tries to fall asleep. He is frustrated that it takes another hour before he actually falls asleep.

Leorra has a stressful semester with a full course load. When she gets into bed and notices that she feels anxious, she tries to relax by shutting her eyes, using relaxation apps, sleeping with a sleep mask on, and taking an antihistamine. Nothing seems to work to help her fall asleep.

Chris brings his laptop to bed with him. He streams programs and has a few favorite websites he visits. He spends a little time on social media sites. He enjoys these activities and is frustrated that he continues to have sleep problems.

Can you identify any possible problems with these wind-down strategies? Do you have any ideas about new things they could try? Let's go through some things to consider in developing a good wind-down routine while considering their experiences.

TROUBLESHOOTING WIND-DOWN ROUTINES THAT DO NOT APPEAR TO BE HELPFUL

Use the form A Closer Look at Your Wind-Down Routine (which you can download at http://www.newharbinger.com/44383) to help you evaluate your wind-down routine. Do you have a specific time during which you start and finish your routine? If the answer is no, and you find that you aren't regularly engaging in your routine, actually having a plan (for example, I will do this one hour before bed) will likely help you engage in your routine more regularly. Can you identify any problems with your routine? Are there too few activities (for example, there is only one activity)? Would it be helpful to add another or even replace it? Is your routine unpleasant? Does it cause you to stay up later (because it is difficult to stop at a good time)? Does it involve your "doing" self or your "being" self? Even if you cannot pinpoint the exact problem (other than that it is not helpful), brainstorm about other activities or how to modify your activity to make it more successful. Make a list and be creative. Pick one or more strategies you want to test this week and keep track of the results. Continue with this process until you are reasonably happy with the result.

At the same online site you will see that there is an example of the wind-down form filled out by Avida. She knows that her current wind-down routine of catching up with friends is causing problems for her, because she can't disengage from her phone. She comes up with some new activities to try, including yoga, a bath instead of a shower, a meditation app, and setting a timer for exiting the chat.

When Avida tried this plan, she struggled, finding it difficult to exit when the alarm went off. So she shifted her whole schedule earlier, hoping that she could exit the chat earlier, and it worked. Although this worked for Avida, many people might have difficulty with this plan out of fear that they might miss out on something as the conversation continues without them.

FOMO: FEAR OF MISSING OUT

Avida had considerable difficulty with disengaging from conversations with her friends, because of a fear of missing out. When you log out, the social media world continues to unfold and events continue to happen. When you wake up in the morning, you may discover that lots has transpired since you were asleep, and perhaps you are disappointed that you were not on social media as it was happening. The benefit of staying online is that you see events unfold live. But you cannot experience every event on social media live—you are, in fact, always missing out on something.

If you suffer from FOMO, it is important that you carefully consider the costs associated with FOMO-driven behavior. Because it is impossible *not* to miss out on some things, this leads to constant disappointment, as well as increased anxiety and depression. FOMO increases your social media time, which tends to result in later bedtimes, less sleep, less physical activity, lower grades, lowered self-esteem, increased depression and anxiety, and (ironically) increased social isolation.

FOMO is a problem independent of sleep, and if it is having a negative impact on your life it is worthy of your attention. Try an experiment in which you take a break from social media for a particular amount of time. Decide on a duration and stick to it—for example, five days. Journal during this period. What purpose did your time on social media serve for you? Can you get this need met in another way? Track what you learn and what you gain from taking the break, and track your sleep during this time. A break of 14 days (or 7 days minimum) would provide the clearest picture of the effect your social media break has on your sleep.

Your social media use can serve as a distraction from anxiety or depression, or other difficult emotions and thoughts. The problem is that increased social media use actually increases those experiences. If you suspect this is the case, try an alternative engaged coping strategy, such as mindfulness or relaxation techniques (covered in the next chapter). Brainstorm other activities that can serve the same purpose. Most importantly, it may be time to consider getting additional support or treatment for anxiety and depression. See the online "Suggested Readings and Resources" (http://www.new harbinger.com/44383) to find help that suits your needs.

"TRYING" TO SLEEP, AND OTHER UNHELPFUL HABITS

What if I were to offer you a million dollars to fall asleep right away? Could you do it? If you have insomnia, probably not. The problem is not about motivation A million dollars would certainly provide high motivation to fall asleep. But if I were to make you this offer, it would increase the pressure to sleep and, ironically, make it more difficult to fall asleep. Falling asleep is like falling in love—it must unfold naturally. Efforts to make it happen will not work, and may even make it worse, as we saw in the above example of Leorra.

USE ANXIETY-MANAGEMENT STRATEGIES

It is important to note that a wind-down routine is about transitioning from your wakeful, alert, problem-solving, "doing" self into a "being" self. It is about setting the stage for the next act—sleep. That said, sometimes it is not enough to have transition activities, and anxiety management is needed. If you are experimenting with activities and your wind-down routine isn't producing the results you want, consider adding a relaxation strategy to your evening. These techniques are covered in detail in Tip 4, but briefly, breathing, mental imagery, progressive muscle relaxation, yoga, and mindfulness exercises can be helpful additions to your wind-down routine.

WIND DOWN OUTSIDE OF BED, NOT IN BED

As important as a wind-down routine is, it is important to protect your bed's status as "The Place Where You Sleep." What does this mean? Think about the example of Chris, above. Chris is engaging in enjoyable activities on his laptop, but this is done in bed, and Chris is frustrated that it takes so long to fall asleep. If you do activities that you do while awake while you are in bed, you may be training yourself to be awake in bed at night. Winding down implies that you are awake, and it is better not to do wakeful activities in bed. Wind down outside of the bed and then get into bed once you feel sleepy. Remember, sleepy doesn't mean tired (see Tip 5); it means that you are about to fall asleep. Signs of sleepiness include noticing that your eyes are rolling back in your head, your head is falling forward or snapping back, you have to reread the same page or rewind a scene you are watching—in short, signs that you are in the process of falling asleep. These are signs that you should stop your wind-down routine and go to bed.

Some people have good wind-down routines only to find that as soon as they get into bed, they become wide awake. Does this sound like you? I call it the "switch" story. The idea is that getting into the bed is like turning on a switch, and you are left feeling wide awake. If you go to bed and notice that you are wide awake, it is a sign that your bed has become associated with being awake. This happens either because when you do wakeful activities in bed the association of the bed with sleep weakens, or because you have had an extended sleep problem that entails lying awake in bed. In either case, if you get into bed and it is like a switch was turned on, and you are now wide awake, it means your bed has become the place for wakefulness.

The way to retrain the brain into thinking of the bed as the place to sleep is to reserve the bed only for sleep. If you notice you are awake and suspect that sleep is not going to happen any time soon, it is important to give up the effort to "try to sleep." Normally we would ask people to leave the bed and the bedroom if they cannot sleep, but this recommendation can be tricky with teens, who often spend too little time in bed and who can become overly activated by activities once they leave the bedroom. If you leave the room, experiment with activities that do not become so interesting and stimulating that you spend hours awake and out of the bed. Your goal is to pass the time out of bed and wait for the sleepiness feeling to return. The return of sleepiness is your cue to get back into bed.

If you are someone who gets excited about activities and finds it difficult to break away from these activities, or if getting out of bed creates conflict with your parents, who would prefer that you rest instead, an alternative is to give up the effort to sleep, sit up in your bed, and do something nonstimulating until sleepiness returns. You can do almost anything that doesn't suck you in to greater wakefulness. For example, many teens like to start texting their friends to see if they are awake, but your friend could say something upsetting or exciting that makes you feel more awake and the act of waiting for their text, thinking of a reply, typing it, and then waiting for their response takes a fair amount of alertness. Picking a low-stimulation activity is key.

Summary

- If you do not have a routine, you should try to establish one. In making a new routine, avoid activities (1) that are too engaging to easily stop, (2) that are done with bright lights, (3) that could lead to charged emotions, and (4) that are done in bed.

- When testing a new routine or activity within your routine, you should notice less alertness right before bed, but on the Tracker or the DOZe app you should also see a decrease in the average time to fall asleep. If you don't notice these two things, keep experimenting with other wind-down activities.

- Wind-down activities are *not* about trying to bring about sleep, because this typically backfires. Wind-down activities set the stage for a state that is compatible with later sleep.

- Sometimes anxiety-management activities are needed in your wind-down routine, if your routine isn't giving you the results you desire.

Your Plan for the Week

☐ Write down your current wind-down routine to determine if anything should be changed.

☐ If you do not have a wind-down routine, generate a list of possible wind-down activities to try this week.

☐ Pick at least one new activity to test as a wind-down. Track the time it takes to fall asleep using the Sleep Tracker or the DOZe app.

Make a Plan for Managing Anxiety

People with insomnia say the number-one reason they have trouble falling asleep is that they feel anxious or have anxious thoughts right before bed. Anxiety is experienced in many different ways, such as feeling scared or tense or worried, or having an upset stomach or chronic muscle tension. You may not think you have anxiety, but if you have headaches or sore muscles or a sore jaw for no particular reason, you should be aware that these are common complaints of people with underlying anxiety. We know that if you feel anxious, it will take longer to fall asleep and you may have poor sleep throughout the night. We also know that if you have poor sleep, you are more likely to have increased anxiety and tension the next day. But the good news is that if you use anxiety-management techniques, your sleep improves, and if you improve your sleep, your anxiety lessens. The bottom line is that there is hope for improving both sleep and anxiety. In this chapter you will learn proven techniques for relaxation, including being aware of anxious thoughts, breathing easier, taking a mental vacation, incorporating more play into your day, and becoming more mindful.

The Case of Arianna and Her Struggles with Unwanted Negative Thoughts

Every evening, as her bedtime approached, Arianna began to think about things that could go wrong the next day or things that she had done during the day that she regretted or felt bad about. The more she had thoughts about feeling nervous or bad about her choices that day, the more upset she felt. The more upset she felt, the less "prepared" she felt emotionally to go to sleep. Having unwanted, repeated negative thoughts like this feels like being on a never-ending Ferris wheel—a Ferris wheel that gains momentum and continues to run on negative emotion. Ariana wanted a strategy to get off the Ferris wheel, and she asked her counselor about it. The counselor asked Arianna to keep track of what was keeping her from getting to sleep, to see if they could identify any patterns. The counselor asked her to track:

- *The situations that sparked a problem for her before bed.*

- *What thoughts she noticed.*

- *How the thoughts made her feel.*

- *The result of the situation-thought-emotion sequence.*

After keeping track of these patterns for a week, Arianna noticed when she was streaming shows at night, her mind would wander to worry thoughts like, "I am going to flub that presentation tomorrow." Arianna noticed that when this happened, the result was more negative thoughts about possible disasters the next day, and she also noticed that she would start to feel anxious. When Arianna felt anxious, she had a tightness in her chest, her stomach felt unsettled, and her breathing was faster than normal. She also noticed that when she felt anxious, the negative, worry-related thoughts became even more anxiety-provoking and more difficult to ignore. She noticed the same pattern with thoughts about choices she regretted during the day (that is, self-critical thoughts) and feeling sad or angry at herself. That is, she would have a thought like, "I can't believe I spilled my drink all over Christine. I'll bet everyone thinks I'm a klutz. I am never going to have any friends."

Arianna is someone who would likely benefit from trying some of the anxiety tools in this chapter, but how about you? Is anxiety a problem for you?

SELF-TEST: COULD A RELAXATION PRACTICE BE HELPFUL FOR YOU?

Not everyone with a sleep problem has an anxiety problem, so let's see if the tips in this chapter could be useful to you. Which of the following apply to you?

- ☐ You feel anxious/tense/agitated/worried in the time leading up to bedtime.

- ☐ You feel anxious/tense/agitated/worried in bed.

- ☐ You feel anxious/tense/agitated/worried throughout the day.

If any of these apply to you, you may find it helpful to use this chapter. Even if you do not have problems with anxiety, many of the techniques in this chapter help people feel more focused and have more energy for their day.

MOUNTAINS VERSUS MOLEHILLS

The way we think has a large impact on how we feel, and changing the way we think about something can change how we feel. You can see how Arianna's thoughts made her feel more anxious, which made her thoughts more anxious, and so on. Being nervous or anxious is a normal part of the human experience. In fact, it is really important that we experience anxiety from time to time in order to deal with actual threats. It is important not to see anxiety as something terrible. The more you want to avoid the experience of anxiety, the more anxious you become about anxiety, and the more anxious you will feel. There is an old saying, "Don't make mountains out of molehills." Molehill thoughts are realistic thoughts about the actual amount of risk and fear appropriate to a situation. Mountain thoughts are negative anxious thoughts out of proportion to the actual situation. Mountain thoughts are like gasoline for your anxiety fire. Given the exact same scenario, which thought would be associated with more post-thought anxiety?

Mountain thought: "OMG, this is going to be a disaster."

Molehill thought: "This may be tough; I should think of something to manage this."

Molehill thoughts are more likely to be associated with using a strategy like taking a moment to slow your breathing, asking for help, or using visualization. Mountain thoughts are associated with increased negative thoughts and anxiety, as well as little action to help manage whatever the problem is. As the old saying goes, it's okay for you to have butterflies in your stomach—just make the butterflies fly in formation. What this means is that anxiety can be used as something positive: as a way to keep us alert and safe or to provide a competitive or creative edge while performing. It is only when you feel excessively anxious (that is, much more anxious than the situation warrants) or it keeps you from doing the things you need to do (for example, sleep) that a relaxation strategy is important to try.

"I'VE TRIED TO RELAX, BUT IT DOESN'T WORK"

If you have tried something that helped manage anxiety in the past, I would suggest that you start using that strategy again. However, you may have had a negative experience with relaxation suggestions, which can be frustrating. The good news is that one method is not invariably superior to another, so try out new ones that work better for you. Relaxation can be used as an in-the-moment strategy, but most techniques require practice until they can be used in an anxious situation. Pick from the menu of relaxation strategies below.

MINDFULNESS

You have probably heard about "mindfulness," but what is it? There are many ways to define mindfulness, but for our purposes we can think of it as taking time to direct your attention in a particular way. The act of directing your attention *toward* something often results in directing your attention *away* from something else that is unhelpful.

Let's think about Arianna. While streaming at night, Arianna's attention became focused on thoughts that made her feel upset, but although she wanted to stop thinking about these thoughts, telling herself to stop thinking about them was not helpful. Telling yourself to "stop thinking" about something is often not helpful because attention remains focused on that thing. But there is a different way to use your attention so that it breaks the thought-distress cycle.

Dr. Jon Kabat-Zinn is one of the leading figures in mindfulness, and he famously said that starting a mindfulness practice is like weaving a parachute—it takes a long time and you don't want to start weaving your parachute after you jump out of a plane. Too often, we are tempted to use a relaxation strategy only when we are very anxious or upset, and it is very hard to use the tool under those circumstances. Instead, try a mindfulness exercise for a few minutes every day and your parachute will be ready when you need to use it. Below are three mindfulness exercises you can try this week: mindful breathing, doing an activity mindfully, and mindfully engaging your senses.

Pay Attention to Your Breath

For this exercise, you are going to pay attention to your breath only. Your mind will likely wander away from your breath from time to time, and that is okay—this exercise is not about keeping your mind perfectly on the breath; it is about noticing when it wanders, and gently returning your attention to the breath.

Find a comfortable sitting position for this exercise. If you are concerned about time, you can set a five-minute alarm on your phone, so that you can set it and forget it. Once you are comfortable, close your eyes softly. It is not necessary to close your eyes, but having fewer (visual) distractions may make it easier. You should be breathing normally, comfortably. Direct your attention to your breathing. What do you notice on the inhale? Air is passing your nostrils, up into your nose. What do you notice about how this feels? Do you feel a slight vibration? Warmth? Perhaps you are breathing in through your mouth. What do you notice about the breath passing over your lips, past your teeth, over your tongue, and down toward the back of your mouth and into your throat? Now the breath is in your chest: does it feel warm? Did your chest expand? Did your diaphragm expand or contract? What did that feel like? The breath is going to leave your body now; what do you notice? Is there a sound? What are the sensations? Is your chest expanding or contracting? What about your belly? What does the breath feel like as it escapes from your mouth or nose? Spend five minutes paying attention to the breath. Nonjudgmentally acknowledge any distraction away from the breath and gently return to the breath again.

Much of the repetitive thinking that perpetuates a negative mood and upsets us tends to be based in the future (for example, What if [something bad] happens?) or in the past (for example, Why did I do that? I feel so [embarrassed/guilty/worthless]). There is nothing you can do to change the past, because it has already occurred, and there is nothing you can do about the future, since it hasn't happened yet. The present moment offers some peace and an opportunity to pay attention to thoughts other than the most distressing thoughts.

Mindfulness is a skill that needs to be practiced. The more you practice, the easier it becomes, and the more results you will see, so I encourage you to start practicing this week.

Do an Activity Mindfully Each Day

One way to practice mindfulness is to schedule one activity a day, and do it mindfully. It can be anything. For example, take a mindful walk. Pay attention to every step on your walk, your breathing, your environment, the temperature, the sounds. Many people say that this is like going to a new place. You can notice something new about a route you have taken a million times before, just by slowing down and paying attention. Stop. Look up. What do you notice? What do you notice about the sound of your footsteps, or about your shadow? It's okay if your mind wanders from paying attention to your walk—simply bring it back without criticizing yourself. Bring your attention back as many times as you need to.

Another activity you can do mindfully is to do a mindful task. If you are doing a chore you don't want to do, such as doing the dishes or the laundry, slow down, do it mindfully, and notice how it may seem different. Every day, pick a new activity to do mindfully. Just remember to start with a breath, direct your attention to the experience, and nonjudgmentally bring your attention back to the experience when you notice your mind has wandered.

Mindfully Engage Your Senses

You might also consider a mindful activity that engages your senses of smell, taste, sight, hearing, and touch. Set aside a particular amount of time, perhaps start with two minutes, and take in your immediate environment with your senses. When you choose to do this activity, there will be no impending disasters to worry about, you are in the here and now, and it is your chance to connect with the perfectness of the present moment.

Smell. Take in the smell of a flower. What do you notice? Really concentrate on the smell of the flower, and notice if there are other smells in the same area as the flower. Does the smell of the flower change subtly as you move farther away or get closer to the flower? Become curious. Become a super smeller and when your mind wanders, notice that and nonjudgmentally bring it back to the smell. Use whatever smell in your environment that you like.

Taste. Mindful eating is a common beginner practice when people are first learning about mindfulness. We often eat mindlessly—shoveling food into our mouth, not noticing the taste or paying attention to satiety cues that tell us we are full and should probably stop eating. Instead, take a piece of food, hold it to your lips, imagine what it will taste like, and take your time as you slowly part your lips, preparing to place the food in your mouth. If your mind wanders, gently notice that your thoughts have wandered and direct your attention back to the piece of food. Let the tip of your tongue touch the food. What do you notice? When you are ready, place the food on your tongue. What does it taste like? What do your tongue and mouth do in response to the food being on your tongue? Pay attention to where the food gets shifted as your mouth prepares to bite the piece of food. Take your time to notice what is happening in your mouth—the taste, the movement, salivation, swallowing. Continue to pay attention until the one morsel of food is completely gone.

Sight. Find something of visual interest and slowly spend time scanning over the sight. Perhaps it's a painting. Perhaps it is a closer look at blades of grass or clouds in the sky. Anything can be visually interesting when we slow down to take in the visual features of the scene or object: colors, textures, patterns, foreground, background. Take it all in. If you notice your mind wandering, it's okay—simply bring your attention back to the visual item or scene. This exercise may amaze you. Young adults have such incredible access to massive amounts of visual information that they are accustomed to scanning quickly. Slowing down and paying attention will open your experience up to new, amazing things. Directing your attention is a practice that also helps with managing strong emotions and unwanted thoughts, as well as with health and well-being.

Sound. Paying attention to the breath involves mindful listening, as we tend to focus on the sound of the breath, but there are other ways to engage hearing to bring yourself to the present moment and your immediate surroundings. Simply close your eyes and listen to what you can hear. Try to identify at least three sounds in the room. It is often surprising how many sounds occur in a room when we are usually oblivious to their presence.

Touch. There are so many opportunities to do a mindful activity wherein you can focus on how something feels. A common activity is to take a warm shower and focus your attention on the water hitting your body. Start the shower before getting in so that it is a desirable temperature. Take a deep breath and step into the shower. (Baths are good for this exercise too.) Focus attention on the temperature of the water and perhaps the variations in temperature as the water runs off your body. When you soap up your body, pay attention to the feel of the bubbles and the way the soap and bubbles feel on the different contours of your skin. Many people set aside their shower (or bath) as their time for a meditation practice every day. It is a solitary activity, done every day, and it has lots to pay attention to. Combining all these sense-related mindful activities can provide a rich opportunity to focus your attention on the present moment. How does the water feel? What scents are you aware of? Breathe deeply and pay attention to the smells of soaps and other products, or perhaps just the smell of the fresh clean shower. What are the sounds in the shower? Follow the sight of the bubbles as they roll off your body and make their way to the drain. Take in everything and gently redirect your attention to the present experience when your attention wanders off the task.

TAKE A CALMING BREATH

There isn't really one method of breathing that is right for everyone as a strategy, but breathing slowly tends to calm people down because it sends a message to the brain that there is no emergency at hand. Arianna could benefit from this strategy by taking a moment when she notices anxiety to slow down her breathing. Sometimes the pace of your breathing can make you feel anxious, so if this is the case, adjust your breathing to something that feels better suited to you. Here are two methods to try: the One-Two-Three Method and the Four-Seven-Eight Method. Try them both and see which one you like better. You can track your results on the Relaxation Practice Log (which you can download at http://www.newharbinger. com/44383). This log tracks the number of minutes and number of times you practiced a particular relaxation tool, and it will also remind you of your goal for the week. It also enables you to track your level of tension before and after the exercise, which allows you to see changes within your relaxation session, as well as your level of tension over time.

The One-Two-Three Method

This method is as simple as taking a long breath in through your nose for a slow count of three. To ensure you are not breathing too rapidly, some people like to insert a silently pronounced word inside each count, such as "one Mississippi, two Mississippi, three Mississippi." As you take the breath in for a count of three, your lower lungs should fill first, followed by your upper lungs. Now hold this breath in your lungs for the same slow count of three. Feel the warm sensation in your expansive lungs. Then exhale very slowly through pursed lips for the same slow count of three. While you are exhaling through your lips, relax the muscles in your face, jaw, shoulders, and stomach. Feel those areas drop into a more comfortable position. Continue this exercise for a minute. This exercise can also be done in a situation in which you feel anxious and need to center yourself. Slowing down your breathing sends a message to your body that you are in a more relaxed state, so other anxiety symptoms will decrease too.

The Four-Seven-Eight Method

This method is the same as the one above except the counts are different. Start by exhaling completely through your mouth, making an exaggerated exhalation sound (such as a "whoosh" sound). Now, inhale through your nose for a slow count of four. You are going to hold your breath, just like the first exercise, but this is for a much longer count of seven. After seven seconds of holding the breath in your expanded lungs, exhale through your mouth slowly for a count of eight. Again, making a whoosh sound helps make the exhale long, steady, and complete.

TAKE A MENTAL VACATION

Vacations are a powerful way to take a break from the stress of your life and recharge, to do something exciting, or to just relax. If you could bottle the feeling of a vacation, it would be a very powerful stress-management tool. Even if you have never been on a vacation, try to think of a place you have been, or a place you have seen, in which you felt serene and calm. Your nervous system can experience the same sensations you feel in that place if you practice using your imagination to mentally revisit that place. In other words, using your imagination can give you a mental break from feeling anxious. Teens also report using this technique to help them feel more confident and prepared before tests, job interviews, or sporting events.

To get started, find a private space and get comfortable. Most relaxation techniques are signaled by taking a deep breath and then closing your eyes comfortably. When you feel ready, imagine a scene, wherever you want. The scene should be ideal. It could be a place you have always wanted to visit or a place you have been that was calm and beautiful. It might be a fantasy world with anything you could want. Many people pick serene locales such as beaches, mountains, a lush forest, or a beautiful field, but if these locations do not evoke a sense of pleasure and calm, keep searching your imagination patiently for a scene that works well for you. Enjoy scanning through your imagination for a scene that brings you a feeling of calm. Try not to rush it or feel frustrated if it takes some time to settle on a scene. Imagine all the aspects of the scene, such as the smells, the sounds, the colors, the textures, the temperature, and the points where the environment touches your body.

Take your time to imagine the scene, and you in it, as vividly as you can. If your mind wanders, gently bring it back to your happy scene. In addition to the sensations of the scene, imagine a feeling of being calm and relaxed. Smile softly as you imagine your scene and imagine how pleasant it feels. You can stay in your scene for as long as you want. You can return to your scene, or other scenes that bring you joy, whenever you want. Most people spend five to fifteen minutes in a visualization exercise, but at certain stressful points in your day you may want to find a private place and take just a minute or two to go on your mental vacation.

TEACH YOUR MUSCLES TO RELAX WITH THE TENSE-AND-RELEASE METHOD

As with any relaxation practice, start by finding a comfortable position, either seated or lying down. Take a deep breath, hold it for a few moments, and then slowly exhale. Prepare your mind for a practice focused only in the here and now. Over time you will be able to merely scan your body for tension and then release the tension in that area. But for now, you are devoting this time to paying attention to your body and observing the sensations of tensing muscle groups and feeling the release of the tension in the same muscle groups. You will likely notice on your Relaxation Practice Log that the number of minutes you engage in this practice will decrease over time as you become more adept at detecting, tensing, and releasing relevant muscle groups.

Once you are in a comfortable position, close your eyes, and bring your awareness to your right foot. Tense the muscles in your foot by pointing and curling your toes as you turn your foot inward. Hold the tension in your foot. Notice how it feels to tense your entire foot (hold for about 10 seconds). Now, as you release the tension and relax your foot, focus all of your attention on the sensation of the release of this tension. Notice how different it feels from when the muscles in your foot were tensed. Let it relax as deeply as you are able. Take 15 seconds to continue focusing on the different sensation now that you have released the tension. After 15 seconds, move on to the other foot and repeat the steps. Once you have tensed and relaxed both feet, pause for 15 seconds and move on to your calf.

Bring your awareness to your right calf (the muscles in your lower leg). Tense these muscles by pointing your toes toward your head and notice how it feels when the calf is tensed. Now hold the muscle tension and your focus on this area for 10 seconds. Relax your calf and notice the difference in sensation from when the muscles were tensed. Focus your awareness on how relaxed the calf feels in comparison to when it was tense, then, when you are ready, bring your attention to your left calf and repeat the entire process.

After that, bring your attention to your right upper leg. To tense these muscles, you can straighten your leg and at the same time try to bend your leg at the knee—but do not actually move your leg. Focus on the opposing actions of the two muscles working against each other. If your muscles cramp or spasm during any of the tension components of this exercise, you are exerting too much force—just try to produce some tension. Focus on the tension in your upper leg and thigh. Notice the tightness in your leg muscles and hold for 10 seconds. Now release the tension in your upper leg and focus on the sensation of release. Notice how different your leg feels as you relax it. Let it relax very deeply and when it feels very relaxed, pause for about 15 seconds and then repeat the process for your left thigh.

Now turn your attention to your hip and glute muscles (your butt, your backside, or whatever you call it). Flex your muscles and the sides of your hips. Focus your attention on this part of the body and the sensation produced by the flexing. If you are able, hold the tension for at least 10 seconds. Now focus your attention on the release of these muscles. Notice the difference in sensation between the tension and the release. Focus your attention on this part of your body for at least 15 more seconds.

Now focus on your stomach area. You can tense your stomach muscles by making your stomach as hard as you can. Try and hold the tension for at least 10 seconds. Now, relax your stomach and notice the release of air from your stomach region and the release of your stomach muscles. Notice the difference between tension and relaxation as you let go of the tension in your stomach.

Now focus your attention on the muscles in your upper torso. You can tense these muscles by inhaling and pulling your shoulder blades together. Do not exert too much force. Notice how it feels when your upper back and shoulders are tensed. Hold it for 10 seconds. Now exhale and release those muscles. Let go of all of the tension and notice how different that feels.

Now focus your attention on your upper right arm. Tense this area by bending your arm at the elbow and bringing your hand up toward your shoulder. Tense your bicep and study how the tension feels. Hold this tension for about 10 seconds. Now release the tension and notice how different the tension and relaxation feel.

Now move your attention a little farther down your arm to the muscles in your hand and forearm. You can tighten these muscles by making a tight fist and holding it. Focus your attention on how the tension feels in this area of your body. After about 10 seconds, relax your hand and forearm by opening your fist and letting your fingers unfurl effortlessly. As you do so, notice the sensations in your hand

and forearm. Notice how the tension feels different from the relaxation. Repeat this with your left arm and hand.

Now move on to your neck. You can tense your neck muscles by gently pulling your chin toward your chest and at the same time keep it from touching your chest. Hold this tension for about 10 seconds and focus all of your attention on the sensation of tension in your neck. Now release your neck muscles and focus your attention on the sensation of release. If you are lying down, allow your head to gently sink back into the floor, releasing all tension in your neck. Notice the difference between the sensations of relaxation and tension.

Now move on to your face. You can tense the muscles of your lower face by biting down and, at the same time, pulling back the corners of your mouth. Hold the tension for at least 10 seconds and really focus on how it feels to tighten these muscles. Now, as you relax the muscles and allow the corners of your mouth to fall forward, notice the difference between tension and relaxation. Continue to focus for another 15 seconds on the relaxed muscles of your lower face. It does not matter if your face is 100% relaxed. It is more important to notice the difference between tension and relaxation and focus on the sensation of release. In time and with practice, your relaxation will deepen.

Now focus your attention on the muscles in the central part of your face. You can tense these muscles by squinting (narrowing your eyes) as tightly as you can and simultaneously wrinkling your nose. Tense these muscles now, focusing on how the tension feels. Feel the tightness and hold for 10 seconds. Now let go of the tension in your face. Notice how it feels to release the tension and allow your eye muscles to soften and fall back into place, and the sides of your nose to soften and fall back into a relaxed state.

Lastly, focus on the muscles in your upper face. You can tense these muscles by raising your eyebrows as high as possible. Feel the tightness in your upper face and focus on this sensation for about 10 seconds. Now, relax your upper face. Let your eyebrows drop and feel the tension releasing from this area.

This exercise takes about 20 minutes. If you are able to commit to trying it daily for a week, you should notice an improvement in being able to target areas of tension for release, and perhaps even in your ability to sleep better.

PLAY EVERY DAY

As we get older, we tend to forget about the importance of physical activity and think of physical play as something for little kids. But physical play (such as sports or dancing) is also important for the health and well-being of adults. When you think of relaxation, you might think that being physically active seems counterintuitive, but expending energy can often help burn off nervous energy. There are many teens who do not like the inactivity associated with formal relaxation, so activities like yoga or sports can be a good alternative. When you engage in sports, your attention switches to the game at hand, redirecting unwanted mental activity. Physical activity also releases muscle tension, increases blood flow, and reduces tension. Most people also find it rewarding to play and it tends to be a social event, so there are many advantages to exercising. What you do when exercising may not matter. Try out different activities and test whether they are helpful for you. Physical activity also has a positive impact on sleep, as it builds the drive for deep sleep.

TRY A YOGA POSE

Yoga has been tested as an insomnia treatment with some positive results. A yoga practice encourages you to slow down your breath and focus your attention on your body and the present moment. There are many forms of yoga; some forms focus on energizing which you may want to do during the day, but for now, let's focus on a relaxation-based practice. There are classes at gyms or at community centers, as well as many YouTube and other online resources where you can learn yoga tailored to young adults. Additionally, there are Instagram accounts of teens and young adults who share their practice via their account. I encourage you to try different resources and find something that appeals to you, but if you want to do something right away, here is a pose to try.

Lay Down Daily for Relaxation

Many yoga practices close with the *savasana* pose. The savasana pose is also called the corpse pose. As with all yoga poses, it is important that you approach yoga nonjudgmentally. There is no "perfect" pose. There should only be your engagement with the pose in the perfect present moment. Set aside 5 minutes to do this pose. Set a timer on your phone so that you don't have to keep looking at the phone or a clock. Sit down on the floor with your knees bent and your feet on the floor. Slow down your breathing and lower yourself slowly back onto your elbows on the exhale. Inhale and slowly extend one leg and then the other. Let your feet soften at the ankles and sink toward the floor, creating an evenness in both feet. Sink into the floor and preserve a small arch in your lower back. Broaden your skull on the floor, finding a comfortable resting place for your head. Use a blanket or small pillow if you would prefer. Inhale and stretch your arms up toward the ceiling. Gently rock back and forth to spread your shoulder blades out from the spine. Exhale, and slowly lower your arms to the floor, with the back of your hands on the floor. Spread yourself comfortably on the floor. While slowly breathing, let your tongue, eyes, and forehead soften. Let your eyes and brain sink to the back of your head. Spend the remainder of your time breathing and relaxing into the floor.

Summary

- Anxiety and sleep affect each other, which means that attempts to manage one more effectively can lead to improvements in the other.

- Learning to relax can take time, but it is easily achieved by investing time in a relaxation practice.

- There is no evidence that one relaxation method is superior to another method, so test out which one works best for you. You can use the Relaxation Practice Log to track your progress for the week.

Your Plan for the Week

Pick a relaxation technique to try from the menu below, and track the results on the Relaxation Practice Log:

☐ Deep, paced breathing

☐ Visualization

☐ Progressive muscle relaxation: tense and release

☐ Sports and exercise

☐ Yoga

☐ Mindfulness

Stay Awake During the Day by Addressing Sleepiness

In the previous chapters we focused on simple strategies to help with difficulty falling asleep or staying asleep through the night. But what happens when the problem is sleeping too much or falling asleep during the day? These are problems with "sleepiness," and they are common problems that often get overlooked. This chapter will help you determine the optimal amount of time you should spend in bed, as well as provide tips for managing sleepiness when you are unable to spend the optimal amount of time in bed.

WHAT IS SLEEPINESS?

Sleepiness is the state you feel as you are falling asleep. Your eyes are heavy and beginning to close or roll back in your head, your neck may snap forward or back, you may need to put your head down on the desk, or you may jerk yourself awake, never realizing you had fallen asleep. It's not the same as feeling tired, which is a state of weariness that can happen anytime during the day but that is not necessarily associated with falling asleep.

Sleepiness is a very important cue in your body that is nearly impossible to ignore or even fight off. If you are old enough to drive, sleepiness can be a deadly experience: falling asleep at the wheel claims many lives every year. Sleepiness also makes it difficult to get through a school day effectively. In adulthood, sleepiness is associated with many diseases, including heart disease, stroke, diabetes, and obesity. It is important to learn how to spot and eliminate sleepiness now, so that it doesn't affect your health long term.

UNDERSTAND THE "SLEEPY CYCLE"

You may have trouble sleeping during the week because you have to go to bed earlier than your body would like, and this can result in poor sleep and difficulty staying awake the next day. As discussed in Tip 2, the world of young adults is frequently set up so that they have to go to bed when their body clock tells them to be alert, and as a result they can't fall asleep until much later. When they finally do fall asleep, they are woken up early by an alarm to get ready for school and they feel sleepy and doze all day at school.

To complicate matters, although sleep deprivation and consequent sleepiness during the week is common, on the weekend the problem is the opposite, and parents often complain that young adults sleep "too much." This weekly cycle is a cycle of "skimpy" sleep followed by "bloated" sleep. Complete the test below to see if you have a problem with sleepiness.

Sleepy Assessment

1. During the week, do you:
   - Have trouble going to bed early enough?
   - Have to wake up before you feel you are finished with your sleep cycle?
   - Have difficulty waking up?
   - Have difficulty getting out of bed?
   - Fall asleep through class?
   - Take naps on breaks between classes or when you get home?

2. Do you sleep more than 9 hours on the weekends?

Did you say yes to any of the difficulties or habits listed under 1? Did you say yes to number 2? If so, you are not alone in feeling sleepy. You may try to fill up with extra sleep on the weekends, but most teens find that it doesn't result in feeling any better. If you are tired of this cycle of skimpy sleep during the week followed by bloated weekend sleep, this is something that can be fixed with a few tricks and tweaks. First, let's talk about sleepiness.

USE THE SLEEP TRACKER TO FIX YOUR SLEEPINESS PROBLEM

In the Tip 1 chapter you learned that tracking your sleep and making a two-week change is often all that is needed to see improvements in sleep. I encourage you to complete that two-week step before going on in this chapter, so that you can use some of the numbers here. You can use the numbers from your Sleep Tracker, or from the free DOZe app, to get tailored feedback about your sleep as well as to come up with a plan to sleep better. If you have not completed the Tip 2 chapter, I suggest that you read and complete the exercises there before proceeding to the other chapters in this book. If you choose to read the present chapter first, you can skip the first section, but you may not have a problem with sleepiness, and therefore much of the advice may not actually apply to you.

SLEEPY INDEX ONE: ON AVERAGE, HOW LONG DOES IT TAKE YOU TO FALL ASLEEP?

Is your average time to fall asleep on the Sleep Tracker or DOZe:

1. Between 10 and 30 minutes? If yes, this is a healthy amount of time to fall asleep.

2. Greater than 30 minutes? If yes, sleepiness may not be a problem for you, and you should focus on the insomnia strategies in the book. If falling asleep takes longer than 30 minutes, it suggests you should give up trying to sleep and find something else to do until you become sleepy.

3. Less than 10 minutes? If yes, this is a sign of sleepiness. It means that you are already falling asleep by the time that you get into bed. One night of sleepiness following a night of poor or reduced sleep is normal, as it is the body's way of compensating, but an average time to fall asleep of less than

10 minutes across a two-week period indicates a chronic sleepiness problem that needs to be addressed.

SLEEPY INDEX TWO: ON AVERAGE, HOW MUCH TIME ARE YOU SLEEPING?

The amount of time you sleep naturally varies from night to night. It is recommended that those aged 14–17 years get 8–10 hours of sleep each night. For those aged 18–25 years, the amount of recommended sleep is 7–9 hours. Generally speaking, too little sleep is associated with increased sleepiness, and too much is also problematic (resulting in poorer immunity, diseases, headaches, pain, increased fatigue, and so on). You can determine your total sleep time by subtracting any time that you are awake in bed from your sleep opportunity—in other words, the amount of time that you were in bed for the purposes of sleep. Wakeful time in bed includes (1) the time it took for you to fall asleep, (2) the time you spent awake in the middle of the night, and (3) the time you spent awake in bed in the morning before getting out of bed. You can calculate the average by adding up all the sleep time and dividing it by the number of nights you monitored (ideally two weeks). You can also use the DOZe app, which will automatically calculate all of these indices.

Is your average sleep time:

1. Healthy? (8–10 hours if 14–17 years old; 7–9 hours if 18–25 years old).

2. Too long? (more than 10 hours if 14–17 years old; more than 9 hours if 18–25 years old). If so, experiment with removing

30 minutes from your time in bed on nights in which it is too long. Nights that are characterized by too much sleep should be targeted by setting a wake-up time with an alarm.

3. Too short? (less than 7 hours if 14–17 years old; less than 6 hours if 18–25 years old). There can be a few different reasons for why sleep is too short. One reason is that you have insomnia (that is, you are in bed enough time but you cannot fall asleep or stay asleep easily). If you have insomnia, the solutions that follow this section are not for you. This book is filled with solutions and tips for you, but the problem of falling asleep too quickly and spending too much time asleep while in bed does not apply to you, so go to the next chapter to continue with solutions for your insomnia. The other reason is within your immediate control: you are not spending enough time in bed on sleep-deprived days. If you only spend 6 hours in bed, it is not possible for you to get the amount of sleep you need. The "Solutions for Sleepiness" in the next section will be particularly important for you.

SLEEPY INDEX THREE: ON AVERAGE, HOW MUCH TIME ARE YOU ASLEEP WHILE IN BED?

The efficiency of sleep is measured by calculating the percentage of time that you are asleep while trying to sleep. It is calculated by taking the sleep time and dividing by the sleep opportunity. Generally speaking, you should be sleeping an average of 85–90% of the time that you are attempting to sleep.

Is your average sleep efficiency:

1. Healthy (85–90%)? Under this scenario, on average you are getting relatively healthy amounts of deep sleep, are taking a normal amount of time to fall asleep, and are usually staying asleep.

2. Too low and suggestive of insomnia (less than 85%)? It is possible that you spend *too* much time in bed relative to how much sleep you can produce. If you spend more than 10 hours in bed (or more than 9 hours if you are 18–25 years old), you can experiment with shortening the time in bed by 30 minutes per week to see if you are able to move into the healthy range for efficiency.

3. Too high and suggestive of sleepiness (over 90%)? This means that whenever your body has a chance to sleep, it takes every minute to do so, and this indicates a concerning degree of sleepiness.

SOLUTIONS FOR SLEEPINESS

If you had one or more of the sleepy indices above, consider some changes to address them.

Solution One: Add 30 Minutes to the Time Spent in Bed

If you are not getting enough sleep during the week, you could experiment with adding an additional 30 minutes in bed on the nights when you are getting too little sleep (that is, when your sleep time is low). This will most often apply during school nights. Consider testing whether sleepiness improves by increasing your time spent in bed during the school week. Use the Sleep Tracker to track whether:

- Your sleep efficiency moves into the healthy range (85–90%).

- The time it takes to fall asleep is 10–30 minutes.

- Your weekday naps decrease (since if you are sleeping more, you should have less of a need for a nap).

If increasing your time in bed makes you feel only a little better, take a look to see if you still have a fairly low sleep time relative to what is recommended. If you are still sleeping too little, try adding another 30 minutes, and assess whether you get the improvements you want. You may wonder why I suggest this during the school week only. Typically, you would not set a goal of increasing your time in bed on weekends because most people spend a normal amount or too much time in bed. One way to find out if you should spend more time in bed on the weekend is if your total sleep is below the maximum recommended for your age (that is, you attempt to sleep less than 10.5 hours if you are 14–17 years old or less than 9.5 hours if you are 18–25 years old), but your sleep efficiency on weekend nights is 90% or greater. If so, you could attempt to increase your time in bed by 30 minutes and see if it makes you feel and sleep better

Finding extra time to be in bed can be difficult. There are lots of demands on your time that make it difficult to make extra time. Finding extra time often relates to troubleshooting the following areas. Think about which ones apply to you and try solutions for managing each.

- Understanding and committing to the importance (for your health and how you feel) of putting sleep first.

- Time management. Move things from the morning routine to the evening.

- Winding down earlier, to go to bed earlier.

Solution Two: Keep Your Time in Bed Steady and Healthy

Determining how much time to spend in bed is tricky. You have probably heard about the dangers of too little time in bed. However, too much time in bed leads to problems too. This is counterintuitive, but spending increased time in bed at night or during the day, or being inactive, sends a message to your system that your sleep needs are *less*, so less deep sleep is produced.

Sometimes there is too little time in bed during the school week and too much time on weekends. The goal is to have a similar, regular sleep opportunity for all seven days of the week. Those aged 14–17 are recommended to get 8–10 hours of sleep each night. This means that the amount of time in bed should be a close match (that is, about 30 minutes more than you sleep) to the amount you sleep. For example, it is optimal to spend no less than 8.5 hours and no more than 10–10.5 hours in bed for this age group. For those aged 18–25, the amount of recommended sleep is 7–9 hours, which means that it is optimal to spend no less than 7.5 hours and no more than 9.5 hours in bed for this age group.

Consider testing if sleepiness improves by getting a more stable dose of sleep. In other words, try to spend a similar amount of time in bed on weekdays and weekends this week. You can use the form Is Your Time in Bed in the Healthy Zone? (which you can download at http://www.newharbinger.com/44383). The Healthy Zone is when your time in bed stays from 8.5–10.5 hours. Those who are 18 years and older may be able to spend a little less time in bed (7.5–9.5 hours).

Solution Three: Nap for Sleepiness

Generally speaking, you should have outgrown the need for naps during the day. That said, during periods of sleep deprivation, napping may be necessary to protect against falling asleep involuntarily (that is, while driving or doing something similarly dangerous). Although napping may be necessary as a safety measure or as a way to protect functioning, napping is a sign that there is something wrong with your sleep. Generally speaking, there should be zero minutes of dozing. Dozing is sleepiness, and sleepiness is involuntary falling asleep. Sleepiness while driving is associated with motor vehicle accidents. Sleepiness during class can lead to poor grades. Falling asleep in public is potentially dangerous (for example, someone might take your belongings when you fall asleep on the subway) and socially embarrassing. Sleep should occur only during the sleep period. When it starts to occur during the daytime, it suggests that you are not getting enough sleep or enough quality sleep.

When you are unable to add time in bed during the week, or adding 30 minutes is not enough to address sleepiness, you may benefit from a scheduled nap during the day. If you have a safe, quiet spot where you can nap, ideally in the first half of the day and for less than an hour (to minimize any negative effects on that night's sleep), experiment with whether a nap helps you stay awake during the day. Unless safety is an issue, do not nap on days in which your sleep efficiency from the previous night was normal or low (90% or less), because the negative effects on sleep may outweigh the beneficial effects. Generally speaking, you should not nap on weekends unless your sleep efficiency was normal or low (90% or less). If you are sleepy (that is, you fall asleep unintentionally or you need to take a nap to function), experiment with adding a nap only on days characterized by an objective sign of sleepiness (that is, you fell asleep too fast, you slept "too little," your sleep efficiency was too high, or it feels unsafe or impossible to avoid a nap) to test whether a brief nap helps you stay awake and feel more alert during the day.

Lastly, be sure to keep your eye on safety. If you feel sleepy, do not drive or operate machinery. Take a nap first or find an alternative way to get to your destination. Driving while sleepy is just as dangerous as driving while under the influence of drugs or alcohol.

Solution Four: Don't Underestimate the Role of Sleepiness in Poor Health and Feeling Bad During the Day

What kinds of facts persuade you to make health changes? When teens hear that smoking becomes addictive and that smoking leads to cancer, many will use that information to guide their behavior and opt not to smoke. Others will hear this information and say, "Maybe for other people, but I will be the exception. I won't get addicted and I won't get cancer." This denial of the facts, or "bias toward optimism," is a breeding ground for unhealthy behaviors and risk for serious future consequences, even early death.

Teens are particularly prone to this because one of the last parts of their brains to develop is the part of the brain responsible for seeing future consequences and being able to plan for them adaptively. Many young adults focus on the here and now rather than the future and engage in behaviors and habits that put them in immediate as well as long-range risk for negative events. There are no exceptions to exposure to sleep-loss-related negative health consequences (such as sleepiness, negative mood, impaired memory and concentration, weight gain, and a poor immune system)—just the illusion of escaping the consequences.

Think about any health-related positive behavior you currently engage in (for example, washing hands, wearing sunscreen, drinking water, eating healthy food, or working out) and remind yourself of the reason you are choosing that behavior. Try to apply the same strategy for making healthy sleep choices. Benefits of healthy sleep habits include:

- Feeling more energetic during the day

- Safer driving

- Increased attention

- Improved mood

- Stronger immune system

- Quality sleep

"SLEEPY" SLEEP DISORDERS

Sleepiness can also result from having an undetected sleep disorder. Below are descriptions of sleep disorders associated with sleepiness. If you continue to suffer from sleepiness after implementing the changes in this chapter, or if you can recognize some of the symptoms below in you, talk to your family doctor.

Sleep Apnea

Obstructive sleep apnea is a breathing disorder that occurs during sleep. If you have sleep apnea, you stop breathing for 10 seconds or more many times per hour, every night. While you stop breathing, your brain and the rest of your body are deprived of oxygen. Possible factors for sleep apnea include: (1) loud, nightly snoring, (2) sleepiness, (3) high blood pressure, (4) someone observing you stop breathing while you sleep, (5) a large neck (a neck size of 17 inches or larger for a male, 16 inches or greater for a female), (6) being significantly overweight, and (7) being male. Although sleep apnea is far more common during middle age and older, it is possible to have sleep apnea even as a child. Sleep apnea is very dangerous if left untreated, and it is easily treated with breathing-assistance devices that keep the airway open as you sleep.

Periodic Limb Movement Disorder

Periodic limb movement disorder (PLMD) is a neurological disorder in which the leg twitches, and it creates poor quality sleep. You are probably unaware of the twitches, but if someone has seen your leg twitching and you are sleepy, you should talk to your family doctor. If you have something called restless leg syndrome (RLS), a disorder in which you experience a strong urge to move your legs when at rest in the evening, and you are sleepy, you may want to talk to your family doctor about assessing for PLMD with a night at a sleep lab. Not everyone with RLS has PLMD, but they frequently occur together. RLS and PLMD are treated with medications.

Narcolepsy

Narcolepsy is a neurological disorder in which rapid eye movement (REM) sleep intrudes into wakefulness. Narcolepsy can look differently in different people. Some of the symptoms include (1) "sleep attacks," that is, falling asleep unintentionally throughout the day; (2) cataplexy; (3) hallucinations upon falling asleep or waking up; (4) sleep paralysis; and (5) excessive daytime sleepiness. However, not all of these symptoms have to be present, so narcolepsy can vary from person to person. Cataplexy is a loss of muscle tone in response to something emotional. The loss of tone may result in total collapse onto the floor or a mild buckling of the legs such that the person cannot continue to stand. The head and jaw often slump forward and the arms often collapse to their sides. Common emotional triggers include laughing, being frightened, or being angered. People affected by cataplexy remain aware throughout the attack, which can frighten them and leave them vulnerable to prolonged symptoms. Sleep paralysis is a symptom of narcolepsy (although it can also appear on its own) in which you wake up and briefly are unable to move. This is because paralysis of most major muscle groups occurs in REM sleep and narcolepsy is essentially an intrusion of REM sleep into wakefulness, so the person awakens but has no control over the major muscle groups. Sleep paralysis can occur on its own; in fact, it is somewhat common for young adults to have had this experience at one time or another. When it occurs regularly and with these other symptoms, it is important to determine whether it relates to narcolepsy. The most common treatment approaches involve medication.

Idiopathic Hypersomnia

Another disorder that is diagnosed when you are excessively sleepy (that is, you fall asleep involuntarily during the day) and there is no identifiable cause, is called idiopathic hypersomnia. This essentially means that you are clinically sleepy and doctors are unsure why. This disorder is managed with stimulant medications.

If any of these signs of "sleepy" sleep disorders sound familiar to you, talk to your family doctor.

Summary

- Many young adults are sleepy because they do not spend enough time in bed.

  Tip: Add a half an hour to your time in bed during the week, and use the Sleep Tracker to determine whether you get more sleep and feel better.

- Many young adults have trouble spending enough time in bed during the week because they delay going to bed until very late and then have to wake up early for school.

  Tip: Spend more time in bed by implementing a regular wind-down routine of an hour or more before bed. A time-management strategy of moving tasks from the morning routine to the evening may also be helpful.

- Sleepiness can occur when there are extremes in the time spent in bed on weekdays versus weekends. That is, there may be too little time in bed on weekdays, and too much time on weekends, and neither will make you feel good.

  Tip: Get in the Healthy Zone by creating a stable, regular time in bed that is similar on weekends and weekdays.

- Naps should effectively alleviate sleepiness.

  Tip: If there is evidence of sleepiness, arrange to nap, ideally in the first half of the day and for less than an hour. Napping is not typically needed or advised on weekends.

- Sleepiness can produce unsafe conditions. If you feel sleepy, do not drive or operate machinery.

  Tip: If you are about to drive and feel sleepy, take a nap first or find an alternative way to get to your destination.

- It is possible to experience sleepiness in the absence of any obvious problems (for example, despite the fact that you have an adequate amount of sleep in bed on both weekends and week-days). It is possible that you could have an undiagnosed medical or sleep disorder, and these should be assessed and ruled out.

  Tip: If it is unclear why you are sleepy, it is important to remember that sleepiness can interfere with quality of life and can even be dangerous, so talk about your sleepiness with your family doctor.

Your Plan for the Week

What will be your plan for the week?

☐ No plan. Sleepiness does not appear to be a problem for me. I will read the next chapter.

☐ I will increase my time in bed on weekdays by 30 minutes and track how it feels.

☐ I will use a one-hour wind-down period and limit stimulating activities (devices with blue light, communicating with people who could deliver exciting or upsetting news, gaming, vigorous exercise, and caffeine/smoking/alcohol/marijuana).

☐ To allow for more sleep on weekday mornings, I will move morning activities, such as showering, setting out clothes, packing my school bag, or making lunches, to the evening.

☐ I want to reduce the difference between how much time I spend in bed on weekdays versus weekends this week by keeping my sleep opportunity between _____ and _____ hours.

☐ I will use an alarm to limit how much time in bed I spend on the weekend. If daytime sleepiness is a significant problem for me, I will make a plan for safety, including napping and arranging for someone else to drive.

Develop a Plan for Getting Out of Bed in the Morning

Most young adults complain that they have difficulty getting out of bed in the morning. Difficulty getting out of bed can create conflict for you, as well as negative consequences if you are late for work, school, or other engagements. You may not feel ready to get up at the time at which your alarm is set, and may feel very groggy upon awakening, so that it seems impossible to get up. While there are many obvious reasons why it may be important to get out of bed in the morning, including getting to school or a job, getting out of bed at a regular time also helps with sleep, mood, and alertness in ways you may not have considered.

LINGERING IN THE MORNING: IS IT A PROBLEM FOR YOU?

Does this scenario sound familiar? The alarm sounds in the morning and you don't feel like getting up, so you press the snooze button and it gives you more time to linger or perhaps even to fall back to sleep briefly. This habit results in lingering in bed in the morning past the set rise time. If you regularly linger in bed in the mornings, it would help to see how much you linger. Using the Sleep Tracker or the DOZe app, is there a difference between when you wake up last (item 5) and when you get out of bed (item 6)? If the lingering index from your Sleep Tracker or DOZe is high, it also means that there is time spent in bed while you are still awake. Is this due to hitting the snooze button? Look at the example of Sam's Weekly Sleep Tracker (which you can download at http://www.newharbinger.com/44383). Sam's alarm sounds at 6 a.m. but you can't see this because item 5 captures the last time at which he woke up, which for Sam was 6:30 a.m. There were two snooze activations during this time. When Sam pressed the snooze button again at 6:30 a.m., he remained awake trying to shake off the groggy feeling unsuccessfully. The snooze button was pressed three more times, until finally, at 7:45 a.m., Sam got out of bed. So what's the big deal?

DON'T SNOOZE, OR YOU WILL LOSE

Using the snooze button on an alarm clock has a surprising number of possible negative consequences:

- Prolonged sluggishness in the morning.

- Waking up to the (second) alarm feeling worse.

- Less time during the day to build a drive for deep sleep the following night.

- Increased variability of the time at which you get out of bed, which is associated with jet lag symptoms of fatigue, mental cloudiness, moodiness, and so on.

Your body clock is constantly watching for cues to tell it what time it is, and the time at which you wake up is particularly important for the clock. Providing the clock multiple cues for waking up in one morning, and varying the wake-up time morning to morning with the snooze button, prevents your clock from getting sleepy at the time you want and alert at the time you want.

Stick to a Steady Rise Time to More Easily Rise on Time

Having difficulty getting up at a regular (early) time is made easier by getting up at the exact same time every morning (including on weekends). Getting up at the same (earlier) time shifts your biological clock earlier and will give you stronger alerting signals in the morning. You will also start getting sleepier earlier.

Of course, you could also be such a night owl that it significantly delays the time at which you get sleepy and an early rise time might feel like having to get up in the middle of the night for most other people. You probably have already read Tip 2 about the body clock, so you can refer to that chapter for more details, but briefly, since your body clock is always looking for regular cues to tell it what time it is, the more regular the cues in the environment (that is, you are regular in the timing in which you wake up, get out of bed, get light exposure, eat your first meal, and so on), the more regular the clock will be.

Go to Bed Earlier

Is the problem that you go to bed so late that getting up in the morning becomes more difficult? If so, wind down an hour or so before bed to make it more likely that you will be ready for bed. We have an entire chapter on tips for winding down before bed. If you want to know if this is an issue for you, examine item 2 ("About what time did you turn off the light and try to fall asleep?") on your Sleep Tracker. Look at the downloadable example of Sam's Sleep Tracker information for Monday. He went to bed at 2:15 a.m. but had to wake up at 6:30 a.m. This will not leave enough time for him to get enough sleep. Sam will need to wind down from stimulating activities much earlier in the night to allow for an earlier bedtime.

REARRANGE YOUR EVENINGS AND MORNINGS TO MAKE IT EASIER TO GET OUT OF BED

Sometimes it is so difficult to get out of bed in the morning that the solution is not to try harder to get up earlier—the solution is to get up a little later. Getting up later may seem impossible if you have several things to do in the morning. But a little time management can help you with problems in finding an extra 30 minutes to spend in bed in the morning.

If time management is a problem, you may benefit from the "roll out of bed" technique. That technique involves moving as much of your morning routine to the evening as possible. Move showers, shaving, choosing and laying out clothes, packing lunches and schoolbags, and so on to a time when you have more energy (that is, the evening). Weigh the benefits of having some extra sleep time in the morning with a little extra organization and time in the evening. Try it for a week and see if you like the results.

FEELING AS THOUGH YOU ARE "DRUNK" WHEN YOU WAKE UP

When you wake up, you may experience what we call sleep drunkenness or sleep inertia. This groggy experience includes feeling confused and not wanting to try to get out of bed. There are many unhelpful beliefs people may have about feeling groggy upon awakening, beliefs that can lead to making things worse.

1. Feeling groggy upon awakening is associated with what stage of sleep you were awoken out of. True or false?

True. Some people assume that waking up feeling groggy has something to do with the quality of their sleep, but this grogginess has more to do with the last brain-wave state before awakening (what stage of sleep you were in just prior to waking). When you wake up during a stage of sleep such as REM sleep, you can wake up feeling alert. This is probably why companies have tried to develop and market alarm clock products to wake you up during REM sleep. As appealing as this may sound, it is not advisable to try and find a way to wake up out of REM sleep in order to feel more alert, because ultimately you would end up with less sleep. Instead, focus on accepting the feeling of grogginess as normal, and engaging in some strategies to shake off that feeling more quickly. The presence or severity of grogginess should not be used to determine whether you should get up or stay in bed longer.

2. Feeling groggy upon awakening relates to your sleep quality, so there is nothing you can do to help with how you feel. True or false?

False. Feelings of grogginess pass relatively quickly—usually in 30 minutes, though it may take up to an hour. You can shake off this state more quickly by stimulating your brain with activities that make you feel more alert, such as opening the blinds for bright light, moving, showering, and reminding yourself that how you feel has nothing to do with needing more sleep.

3. The best way to help is to stay in bed and try and get more sleep. True or false?

False. Staying in bed because you are experiencing the normal state of inertia upon awakening can make you feel worse. Even if you wake out of REM sleep on your next awakening and feel more alert, ironically this will have a negative impact on your sleep because it will decrease the amount of sleep you get the next night. Why? Because the amount of deep sleep you produce is directly related to spending increased time active and out of bed. If you increase your time spent in bed, it decreases the amount of deep sleep you will produce. You can shake off grogginess more quickly if you stimulate your brain with activities that make you feel more alert. Think of it this way, if you spend all day on the couch, do you feel more alert or sluggish? An object at rest stays at rest. You're the object, so get moving, expose yourself to light, and alertness will follow!

These questions were meant to show you the downside of assuming that feeling groggy upon awakening means that you had a bad sleep or will feel bad for the rest of the day. Actively challenge thoughts that relate to the wrong cause of morning grogginess and it will pass. Assuming that you will feel bad for the rest of the day can become a self-fulfilling prophesy. That is, if you think you will feel bad, it focuses your attention on evidence that confirms that you feel bad. It also increases anxiety, and anxiety symptoms can lead to feeling bad and feeling fatigued—the very thing you wanted to avoid.

COME UP WITH AN OUTSIDE-IN PLAN

When trying to get out of bed, many people are waiting for a feeling of motivation to get out of bed that never actually comes. We call this an inside-out plan: a plan in which we wait for a feeling, in this case motivation to get out of bed, and then we use that feeling to get moving. However, if you are having difficulty with feeling like you want to get up, or something is getting in the way (for example, sleeping through your alarm clock), an inside-out plan might not work well. Here is an alternative. Use an outside-in plan: a plan in which you don't follow a feeling, you instead follow a plan, and rearrange your environment to support your plan. For example, your outside-in plan may be to get up earlier and at a more consistent time, and if you are not going to rely on a feeling, it means you need multiple strategies in place that make it more likely you can follow this plan. Below are a number of strategies you can try that do not rely on following a feeling (which may not come) and make it more likely that you can achieve your goal.

Sound the (Multiple) Alarms

You may be frustrated because you sleep through your alarm clock. You're making an attempt to get up on time, but the plan isn't working.

You may need more than one alarm to sound (for example, one set at one rise time and then the others staggering to sound at subsequent 10-minute intervals), at different places in the room, in order to encourage you to get up to deactivate them. It may help to leave a sticky note on each clock, phone, or device to remind you of your commitment to get up. For example: "DON'T GO BACK TO BED!" If you must peel off the note to disarm the alarm, it may motivate you to get moving toward the bedroom door, rather than back to the bed. You can also record a message as part of the alarm on most smartphones.

Try a New Alarm Clock or Alarm Clock App

There are apps available at the App Store and Google Play that may be more effective than the standard alarms available on your phone. These alarms require that your volume be turned up on your phone and will alarm even when you have turned your phone to silent. There are a variety available, and some are free. Options range from very loud alarms to alarms that mimic emergency alarms, such as fire alarms, military evacuation alarms, or air horns. There are also options for multiple alarms or alarms that must be disarmed in a complicated way (for example, by solving a math problem).

ASK FOR HELP

If sleeping through your alarm is a particularly difficult problem for you, you may want to ask for help from parents, roommates, siblings, girlfriends or boyfriends, and so on. Communicate that you are having trouble with getting up in the morning and are trying out some new plans to make it easier, and ask them if they can wake you up at a certain time if your strategies aren't working. Setting multiple alarms may bring someone else into your room because the alarms may be so loud and persistent. It is important to talk to people who live with you about your plan, to let them know that if they want to deactivate the alarm, you would appreciate it if they helped you get out bed rather than themselves deactivating the alarm. Since the alarm may be bothersome to others, it is important to have good communication to manage conflict. This also means that you may have to commit to trying multiple strategies in this chapter to limit the impact of your sleep difficulties on others living with you.

MAKE A PLAN FOR COMFORT

Imagine that you are warm and comfortable in your bed, with your blanket up under your nose, the tip of your nose is poking out of the blanket, and it is "ice cold." How motivated do you feel to get out of bed? Temperature and comfort matter to people, and can be a factor in not wanting to get out of bed. If this is a factor for you, you can plan to maintain warmth as you transition out of bed.

- Take your blanket with you to a chair in another room. When you feel more alert, you can continue with getting your morning started. As long as you do not lie down, you have met your goal of getting up.

- Keep your favorite socks, slippers, sweats, or hat next to your bed and put them on before getting out of bed. You can transition to a chair in another room until you feel ready to more fully activate.

- You can turn on the shower a minute before you get into it, so that you transition right into a steamy, hot shower.

- Brainstorm about something that would make getting out of bed easier and more comfortable, and try it out this week.

WRITE DOWN SOMETHING YOU CAN LOOK FORWARD TO TOMORROW MORNING

It can be more difficult to feel motivated to get out bed when you cannot think of a good reason to do so. You may feel less motivated to get out of bed for an activity like going to class, but thinking of an activity, such as going for a coffee before class, arranging to meet up with a friend to walk to school, downloading new music for your walk, or going out for a snack or lunch right after class, can combat feelings of not wanting to get up. It helps to make these plans the day before, because it is difficult to think of things to do while you are lying in bed. If it is the weekend, you can plan something enjoyable for the morning. Including someone else in your plans makes it more likely that you will look forward to doing it.

CONSIDERATIONS FOR CHRONIC PAIN, DEPRESSION, AND ANXIETY

When you read the advice above, you may have thought that planning something enjoyable seems impossible when you feel depressed, because nothing feels enjoyable. Or you may have thought, "How am I supposed to get out of bed if everything hurts?" Dealing with conditions like depression, chronic pain, or anxiety can make this advice seem more difficult to follow, but we know that following this advice may be more important for you than any other group of people.

Depression

People with depression tend to be less active and spend more time in bed. Spending less time active and awake in the 24-hour period is associated with less deep sleep, as well as increased fatigue, pain, and depressed mood. The problem is that if you focus on how good it feels to be snuggled in a bed, you might not link the subsequent feelings of depression, pain, fatigue, and sleep difficulties to this behavior.

There are several effective treatments for depression that include a component of increased activity. Many of these treatments involve establishing an earlier rise time. Getting up earlier tends to increase the time spent out of bed and provides an opportunity for more light exposure. It also increases the chances that you may engage in more activities, which tends to make you feel less depressed and less anxious. Doing more provides more opportunity to experience something positive or to interact with someone in a way that can disprove negative thoughts you may have about yourself or your life. Getting up earlier may also cut off excess REM sleep from occurring, since the bulk of REM sleep occurs in the second half of the night. There is something about REM sleep that is associated with increased depression. And in fact, many antidepressant medications decrease the amount of REM sleep you produce.

Chronic Pain

Increased time in bed is also associated with increased pain in those with pain conditions. It can also cause additional problems. For example, increased time at rest shortens muscles so that when they are used, it is painful. Less activity is also associated with a loss of conditioning (that is, being out of shape), and it also decreases the drive for deep sleep (which is contingent on being active and out of bed enough hours). Deep sleep is important for a variety of reasons, but one important reason is that this is the stage that produces growth hormone, a chemical that heals tissue in your body. If you deprive people of deep sleep, they start to complain of aches and pains, even if they normally have no pain. So you can imagine how badly this would feel for those with chronic pain conditions. Although being active and getting out of bed is more difficult with chronic pain, doing so is very important because it helps with sleep as well as with pain improvement.

Anxiety

If you feel overwhelmed, stressed, or anxious, you may crawl into bed and immediately feel comforted. There is an instant reinforcement of the pairing between the bed and relief. Unfortunately, increased time in bed will eventually lead to increased insomnia and the bed will be paired with wakefulness. Moreover, insomnia is associated with increased anxiety, so the situation has now produced increased anxiety and insomnia.

The more you retreat, the more you reinforce the belief that you cannot cope, and the more prone you become to even more anxiety. This is why we say that decreasing anxiety often involves avoiding avoidance. For example, if you are afraid of social situations, keep approaching social situations in a way that is manageable; if you are afraid of spiders, stay in the situation until your fear decreases; if you are feeling overwhelmed, stay engaged, and do not retreat to your bed. It is the retreat and avoidance that makes fears grow.

MEETING GOALS DESPITE DEPRESSION, PAIN, AND ANXIETY

Many people assume that since it feels good to lie in bed in the morning and it feels less good when you first get out of bed, that this somehow means that they need to, or should, stay in bed. You now know that the opposite is true. So it is important not to follow the feeling of wanting to stay in bed, and instead follow a plan to get out of bed. Use the form My Get-Out-of-Bed Plan (which you can download at http://www.newharbinger.com/44383).

The good news is that the strategies in this book work the same for people without problems like depression, pain, and anxiety as they do for those with these problems. However, because it may be more difficult, more strategies need to be used (and written down so that they are remembered) to make success more likely. Trying only one strategy may not be as effective for you.

Write down your plan. It may include (1) reducing your lingering in bed to under 30 minutes during the week; (2) limiting sleeping in to 9 a.m. at the latest on weekends; (3) putting comfortable sweats and slippers by the bed to minimize the shock of cold upon awakening; (4) trying a new alarm; (5) enlisting help; (6) using the roll-out-of-bed technique; (7) taking a warm shower in the morning; (8) opening all the blinds while eating breakfast; and (9) scheduling something rewarding for yourself in the morning. You may not be able to do all of these, but writing down these ideas and keeping them next to your bed may make it more likely for you to be able to reach your goal. Additionally, write some reasons why you are committing to getting up earlier. In the morning, when you feel groggy and may not remember *why* it is important for you to make this change, you will be less likely to commit to doing it.

Lastly, be realistic in what goals you set. Although you may need many strategies to increase the likelihood you can do it, don't set goals that are not possible for you to meet currently. For example, you might decide to shorten your lingering time by 15 minutes per day even though your end goal is to shorten it by one hour. Better to achieve your goal and feel encouraged, than to set too high a goal and feel discouraged or experience harsh self-critical thoughts. Be patient and kind with yourself: it is tough to form new, healthier habits. As with anything in this book, if you are struggling to implement the strategies, don't be afraid to reach out for professional help.

Summary

- Making a change, such as getting out of bed earlier and more regularly, can be difficult, so it's important to try multiple methods to help. Make a list of ideas to try, and track the results this week.

- Getting out of bed at a regular time sets your body clock, and that will make it easier to get out of bed earlier.

- Try the roll-out-of-bed routine to get more sleep and a little extra time in the morning.

- Actively challenge false notions of the cause of morning grogginess.

- Be creative in trying out new alarm clocks, staggered around the room.

- Ask for help as a backup to help you get out of bed.

- Comfort is important. If you are resisting getting up because you don't want to feel cold, make a plan to stay warm (for example, take your blanket with you when you get up, or put on a robe or a sweater).

- While trying to make a steady rise time a habit, plan something special for the morning that you can look forward to.

- Although the strategies in this book work the same for people without problems like depression, pain, and anxiety as they do for people with these problems, struggling with these conditions makes it even more important to use more strategies to achieve your goal of getting out of bed more easily in the morning.

My Plan for This Week

☐ I will try to decrease my lingering-in-bed time. (It's probably best to have a specific length of time in mind, and use the DOZe app or the Sleep Tracker to see if you can do it.)

☐ I will try to maintain a steady rise time (so that my body clock will make it easier to get up subsequently).

☐ I will try to move at least one of my morning routines to the night before and track if this is helpful.

☐ I will eliminate or reduce the use of the snooze feature on my alarm.

☐ If my alarm clock isn't working well, I will try one new method or clock from this chapter.

☐ I will try to shake off morning grogginess by: getting moving right away, turning on bright lights or opening window blinds, or/and taking a shower.

☐ I will schedule one thing to look forward to, at least one morning this week.

Develop a Plan to Feel More Alert During the Day

If you read the chapter on tips to manage sleepiness (Tip 5), you learned that "sleepiness" means that you are actually falling asleep (and quickly). In this chapter, we are focusing not on sleepiness, but on feeling fatigued. Exhaustion, fatigue, weariness, being tired or sluggish—these terms are used interchangeably, and all of them refer to a feeling of depletion or of low energy or motivation. Unlike "sleepy," none of these terms necessarily means that you are actively falling asleep. It is possible to be both fatigued and sleepy, but it is important to know that falling asleep during the day is not a sign of fatigue; it is a sign of sleepiness. This chapter is reserved for the more common daytime experience of fatigue. You will learn whether feeling tired is a problem for you, and tips that manage fatigue, including changing how you think or respond to fatigue, in order to feel more alert.

ARE YOU FATIGUED?

Which of these statements most accurately reflects how fatigued you typically feel?

1. I am rarely tired, and if I am it is an understandable response to overexertion. [score = 0]

2. I am sometimes tired but I can cope easily using some strategies. [score = 1]

3. I am frequently tired most days of the week, or at least half the day, and have to exert effort to perform my daily activities. [score = 2]

4. I am always tired and it affects my ability to perform my daily activities OR I am sometimes tired, but when I am, it is severe and greatly affects my ability to perform my daily activities. [score = 3]

If your score was a 2 or greater, it suggests that fatigue is a significant issue for you, and that learning more about fatigue and how to manage it could be helpful for you. If your score was 0 or 1, your level of tiredness appears to be normal for your age, and if you do experience fatigue, you appear to have healthy effective strategies for managing it.

WHY FATIGUE THOUGHTS MATTER

Thoughts often lead to actions that are consistent with those thoughts. An excited thought, such as "I can't wait to go on this roller coaster," is most consistent with going on the ride, and less consistent with walking away from the ride. We tend to act in ways that match our thoughts, which can be unfortunate because thoughts are not facts, and can sometimes lead us down an unhelp-ful path. Consider Thought 1 and Thought 2, below. Which one is more likely to be associated with helpful fatigue management tools? Which one is more likely to be associated with negative emotion, like frustration, anxiety, or depression?

THOUGHT 1: *"I'm so tired that I won't be able to function for the rest of the day."*

THOUGHT 2: *"I'm tired, but it's temporary. What can I do to manage the fatigue until it passes?"*

Thought 1 is an example of a thought that can become a self-fulfilling prophesy. If you assume that because you are tired, you won't be able to function well, you are more likely to be on the lookout for information that confirms that you aren't functioning well. For example, you may notice a mistake you made at school or a symptom like having tired eyes. If you are not scanning for this evi-dence, it is less likely that minor mistakes and tired eyes will be noticed, and this frees you up to function better and to feel better. There is an old saying attributed to Henry Ford that says, "Whether you believe you can or can't, either way, you are right." Thoughts can make things happen; whether that's good or bad is up to you.

What about Thought 2? It starts with the same noticing of feeling tired as you see in Thought 1, but the prediction is more posi-tive and realistic. Fatigue will pass eventually because fatigue comes and goes, so this thought is both helpful and true. More importantly, this thought shifts you into action—to use tools to help you with your fatigue. The first tool for helping with fatigue is to challenge unhelpful thinking about fatigue.

YOU ARE NOT YOUR THOUGHTS

If particular thoughts about feeling tired lead you to do things that make fatigue worse, the first step is to realize that thoughts are just thoughts; thoughts are not facts and you are not your thoughts. The second step is to shift the thought into something that is more helpful and consistent with your goal of feeling better. For example, look at this thought: "I am feeling so tired, I'm never going to be able to do my assignment. I'm going to fail." This type of thought is particularly unhelpful because the negative outcome is exaggerated and is probably not accurate and certainly not helpful. Struggling with an assignment is a fairly normal experience, and assuming that your momentary failure to get everything right is going to result in you failing your class seems unlikely and rather extreme. This kind of worst-case scenario thinking is called *catastrophizing*, and it fuels anxiety. Dialing that thought back will decrease your anxiety and may make it more likely that you can start working effectively on your assignment.

THE FRIEND TEST

One way to challenge catastrophizing is to use the "Friend Test." That is, think about whether you would provide the same interpretation of a situation to a friend. Imagine your friend saying, "I am feeling really tired today." You would not reply: "You're feeling tired? Oh no! You are never going to get your work done properly. You are going to fail!" What are some of the possibilities for your friend?

- The friend will be able to complete the assignment well, for example earning an A or a B.

- The friend will be able to complete the assignment, but may get a lower grade than usual, for example a C.

- The friend will be able to complete the assignment, but may get a very low mark on it, for example a D.

- In an extreme circumstance, the friend may not be able to do the assignment at all and may have to hand it in late with a penalty.

To assume that the absolute worst-case scenario is always the most likely one is inaccurate and not supportive.

At first, it may be difficult to change a catastrophizing thought. I recommend that when you recognize that such a thought is bothering you: (1) stop, (2) breath, (3) write down the thought that is making you most upset, and (4) spend some time asking yourself questions such as:

- Is the thought that's bothering you true 100% of the time? For example, feeling tired now does not mean you can *never* do an assignment. There have been some circumstances (probably many) in which you've managed to do an assignment even though you were tired. So it is not true 100% of the time.

- Does this thought make you feel less confident about whether you can deal with feeling tired? Believing that you cannot work on an assignment when you are tired can lead you to think you are not capable of coping with feeling tired and functioning, and this thought will make you feel more and more anxious whenever you feel tired.

- Does this thought lead you to do things that will make you feel tired or make you sleep less? For example, if you have a thought that you cannot deal with feeling tired so you are going to drink another energy drink, you may feel better initially. However, some teens find it harder to focus when on caffeine. If you need to feel alert for more than a few hours to get the assignment done, you will eventually be dealing with withdrawal symptoms that include feeling even more tired. The energy drink is also going to have a negative impact on your sleep, which can make you feel tired the next day. This one thought has thus led to a behavior that actually makes things worse.

To organize your thoughts and help you challenge thoughts about feeling tired that make you feel worse, try using the Question Your Thought worksheet (which you can download at www.new harbinger.com/44383). Unhelpful thinking can seem like an automatic process. Slowing down and examining thinking takes time at first, but practicing will eventually make helpful thinking more of a habit.

CHALLENGE THE IDEA THAT POOR SLEEP IS ALWAYS THE CAUSE OF FATIGUE

Is fatigue always related to how you slept? This is a complicated question. This belief can lead to problems. Most people assume that having a poor night's sleep means that you will feel tired the next day. Similarly, if you have a good night's sleep, you should not feel fatigued the next day, right? Let's take a closer look at this idea.

You have probably had the experience in which you felt exhausted during the day and thought, "I don't know why I feel so tired…I had a good sleep last night…" How about the reverse? That is, you had poor sleep but were surprised at how good you felt and how well you functioned the next day. We are biased toward remembering and thinking about situations that support the idea that fatigue and sleep are highly related. This is probably because parents often tell us, "You have a big day tomorrow, so you better get a good night's sleep." We tend to assume that a good sleep means that you will not feel tired and this makes for a good day, but this is not necessarily the case. On the other hand, sleep and sleepiness *are* highly related—if you are sleep-deprived you will have trouble with sleepiness (that is, trouble staying awake).

We conducted an experiment in our laboratory in which we gave people a picture of a circle called a pie chart, and we asked people with insomnia to carve up the pie and label the pieces of the pie to correspond to what accounts for their fatigue. What would your pie look like? Draw it out. You can use the resource Considering Causes for Your Fatigue (which you can download at www.newharbinger.com/44383) and look at Patti's example to help. In our experiment, everyone uniformly made no cuts in the pie and instead labeled the entire pie as "sleep." That means that they believed that their fatigue was 100% attributable to their sleep. Does your pie look like that?

We then split the people into two groups. Half of the people were told things that make you feel tired and the other half were told information about sleep. The group that was told all the reasons why we feel tired felt less anxious about their sleep, and they also said they felt less tired after hearing the new information. Patti's filled-in form shows you all the new reasons she was able to generate after learning about common causes for fatigue. The group that was given information about sleep only still felt anxious and tired. What did we learn from this experiment? Knowing there are many reasons you feel tired can make you feel less anxious about your sleeping problem and less anxious about feeling tired. It may also make you feel less tired overall. Could this information help you? Let's consider reasons for feeling tired other than sleep.

ARM YOURSELF WITH KNOWLEDGE ABOUT WHAT CAUSES FATIGUE

If fatigue is not necessarily about sleep, then what causes it? There are countless causes of fatigue. Here are just a few common ones:

- Eating habits: If you skip meals or eat at irregular times, your blood sugar can spike and drop, creating big changes in your energy level. Unhealthy meals or sugary foods or beverages can also create problems with blood sugar, as well as a sluggish feeling.

- Caffeine withdrawal: Several hours after consuming something with caffeine, the body goes into withdrawal and one of the symptoms is fatigue. If you treat fatigue-related withdrawal symptoms with more caffeine, it will temporarily get rid of the withdrawal fatigue, but the withdrawal will occur again several hours later.

- Boredom: Feeling bored or understimulated often co-occurs with fatigue. Changing your activity or surroundings is often enough to alleviate both boredom and fatigue.

- Motivation: When you are faced with a difficult task and you do not want to do it, or you do not believe you will have enough energy to complete it, your experience of fatigue increases. This is something you can test. Take note of your current fatigue level, then look around your environment for a task that you really do not want to do. Now take note of your fatigue level. Do you see how your fatigue increased just thinking about it? If you have a task you do not want to do, you can devise a plan to make it less daunting, and this should help with your fatigue. For example, you can break up the task into smaller parts, take breaks, pair the task with something you enjoy (for example, streaming music or a podcast, or asking a friend to hang out or even help with it), use encouraging self-talk during the task, or plan a reward after the task is done.

- Overexertion: Very high levels of physical exertion, such as high-intensity exercise, can lead to muscle fatigue, so be sure not to overdo it. That said, exercise is a helpful way to combat fatigue, so it is only during extremely intense exercise that you are likely to experience fatigue. Those who exercise usually do not complain about high levels of fatigue because they also experience increased pleasure due to endorphin release, so it best to experiment with what works for you.

- Underactivity: The biggest mistake when it comes to fatigue is to assume that you need to rest in order to increase energy. Although most people think that overactivity is the main culprit for fatigue, sedentary or low levels of activity can be a bigger culprit. If you are feeling tired right now, stand up, do some stretches, and walk around. Why do you feel less fatigued after such a mild increase in activity? Fatigue occurs during overexertion, but also during underexertion. If you have ever spent a totally sedentary day, you know that you end up feeling more tired, not less.

- Stress or anxiety or a depressed mood: Negative moods sap resources and alter the way you think. Negative moods make you feel like you have low personal resources, and your thoughts tend to be consistent with that negative mood. If you frequently have trouble with negative moods, talk to your counselor or doctor. See the "Suggested Readings and Resources" list at http://www.newharbinger.com/44383, which includes apps, web resources, and helplines for managing moods.

- Alcohol or other drugs: Depressant drugs such as alcohol or stimulant drugs such as cocaine can produce fatigue as a direct effect or as an effect of withdrawal. Avoiding these substances can help you avoid the fatigue associated with them.

- Medical conditions (for example, anemia) and medications (for example, chemotherapy) are also sources of fatigue. Consulting with your doctor, or knowing the side effects of medications you take, can help you determine if your fatigue is related to conditions or medications.

FINDING FATIGUE TARGETS IN YOUR SLEEP TRACKER

Look at the sleep data you collected using the Sleep Tracker or the DOZe app. When we ask people to look at their Sleep Tracker information and look for what is making them feel tired, they tend to say things like taking a long time to fall asleep, spending a lot of time awake in the middle of the night, or sleeping a low amount of hours. Now, however, you know that these are not reliable predictors of feeling tired, and that there are several other things on your Tracker that predict fatigue.

- Your *jet-lag-without-travel* indices. You can create jet lag in any of these indices: Use your Sleep Tracker to look at the earliest and latest times at which you went to bed (item 1), attempted to initiate sleep (item 2), woke up for the last time (item 5), and got out of bed (item 6). The difference between the earliest and latest of each particular one of these jet lag indices approximates the number of time zones you crossed without traveling, and how severe your jet lag symptoms will be. For example, if you go to bed at 10 p.m. on some days but go to bed at 1 a.m. on others, that produces jet lag symptoms similar to traveling three time zones. If you wake up at 6 a.m. on some mornings but wake up at 8 a.m. on other mornings, that produces jet lag symptoms similar to traveling two time zones. If any of your indices is 1 hour or greater, you can decrease fatigue by decreasing the variability on that particular index this week. If you download the DOZe app, it will calculate this index as well as the indices below for you.

- Your *lingering-in-bed* index. Using your Sleep Tracker, look at the difference between when you woke up for the last time (item 5) and when you actually got out of bed (item 6). The difference between these times constitutes increases in rest without sleeping. Increased rest increases fatigue. We need rest as part of sleep, but when we have too much rest without sleep it creates increases in fatigue. I know it sounds strange, but if you shorten your morning lingering time, it will create more energy for you. Once you are out of bed, keep yourself moving by turning on lights, showering, and getting your day started.

RIDE OUT THE POST-LUNCH DIP

It's early afternoon and you are sitting in class, and you suddenly feel very exhausted: mentally, physically, and emotionally. Sound familiar? Why do you think this happens? Do you think it's because of what you ate at lunch? Is it because you skipped lunch? Is it because you are bored with class? Is it a sign that your sleep is poor?

Over the next week, keep track of this special period in the early afternoon and notice that there is consistently a slight dip in alertness for about an hour or so. Why? It is true that nutrition and boredom can have an impact on our fatigue levels, but this predictable post-lunch dip is actually related to your body clock. (For more on the body clock, read Tip 2.) Your body clock is responsible for keeping you alert throughout the day, but after lunch there is a slight dip in body temperature that results in us feeling tired temporarily. Riding out the post-lunch dip can simply mean that you accept that it happens and do nothing at all during the time at which you are experiencing it, or you can try some of the suggestions below.

Activate During the Dip

When you feel tired, you don't feel like doing anything, and when you don't feel like doing anything, you will feel more tired. Although it seems intuitive to rest to get energy, it doesn't actually work that way. An object at rest tends to stay at rest. You need to expend some energy to create some energy. The solution, then, is to make a plan to expend some energy during the dip.

- Go for a walk.

- Do something fun.

- Exercise.

- Change your scenery or go to a different room.

- Take a break from your current activity with a new activity.

- Socialize.

Try this for one week and keep track of the improvements in your fatigue level during the dip.

Challenge Reactions to the Post-Lunch Dip

It is not well understood why the post-lunch dip occurs, but it is important for you to know that how you react to it can create thoughts and behaviors that can make things worse. Which of the following reactions could make things worse?

"I'm so tired that I won't be able to make it through the rest of the day."

"I might as well just go home."

"Going to have to load up on energy drinks now."

"Ugh, this sleep problem is ruining my life."

The answer is: all of them. The post-lunch dip happens regardless of whether or not you slept well the night before, and once it passes, there is no reason that you will not return to your pre-lunch level of energy.

Challenging thoughts that ultimately are unhelpful can change how you are feeling. If one thought is associated with more likely positive outcomes, and the other is associated with negative outcomes, then when you experience the negative thought, you can challenge yourself to consider the more positive alterative.

UNHELPFUL THOUGHT: *"I'm going to have to load up on caffeine and energy drinks now."*

CHALLENGE: *"It's going to pass anyway. If I load up on caffeine, I will be faced with a caffeine crash later. I'll try something different and see what happens."*

UNHELPFUL THOUGHT: *"Ugh, this sleep problem is ruining my life."*

CHALLENGE: *"This dip has nothing to do with my sleep. Focusing on how tired I feel is going to make me feel more tired, and focusing on my sleep problem is going to make me feel even more anxious about my sleep. Instead, I'm going to try a strategy to ride out this temporary dip."*

FIGHTING FATIGUE WITH FOUR STRATEGIES

There are four key behaviors you can use to help manage fatigue, without fixing your sleep. You can remember them by being at the "HELM" of your alertness.

Hydrate. Drink water throughout the day. Dehydration can make you feel tired. Many teens drink sugary or caffeinated beverages to manage fatigue, but try to experiment with one week in which you focus on staying hydrated rather than relying on sugary or caffeinated beverages and you will be surprised at the results.

Eat. Have a healthy meal three times per day. Skipping meals or eating junk food creates blood sugar shifts that can make you feel tired. Eating regularly also provides steady input for the body clock, which reduces "jet lag without travel" symptoms.

Light. Exposure to natural blue spectrum light, like sunlight, makes you feel more alert. Unnatural light, from light bulbs, is the next best thing. In the Tip 2 chapter you learned that blue light helps with daytime alertness and sets the stage for a healthy sleep at night. We make sure kids get enough outside playtime, but as we move into early adulthood, this is prioritized less. Get plenty of daylight by incorporating walks to and from school, or during free periods or lunch periods at school, and enjoying leisure outdoor activities on the weekend.

Move. If you feel more tired with low levels of activity, then it makes sense that increasing activity can help with fatigue. Movement and activity make you feel more alert and help manage fatigue. Moving also breaks your boredom. If you are bored, your feelings of fatigue will be intensified. Schedule a quick break and then return to your task. Exercise is a very effective tool when you are feeling tired, but there is a delicate balance in which vigorous exercise can increase fatigue. Find what exercise and intensity works best for you.

YOGA

Exercise and increased activity are effective strategies for fatigue, but have you ever considered yoga? Yoga is helpful for flexibility, fitness, relaxation, and reducing stress, but it can also help people feel energized. There are yoga poses designed to stimulate energy, so experiment with yoga poses by searching on the Internet for energizing poses. Some poses can include:

Mountain Pose: This pose involves standing tall and evenly on both of your feet, which are placed a comfortable distance apart. Inhale slowly and deeply, raising your arms toward the ceiling, palms facing each other. Reach gently to the ceiling through your arms, shoulders, and fingertips and look up gently. After about five deep breaths, exhale slowly and deliberately bring your hands back down by your sides. Many people with difficulty getting out of bed in the morning create a routine in which they get out of bed, turn on the lights, and use mountain pose to create some energy before starting their day.

Cobra Pose: Find a comfortable place on the floor. Lie on your stomach and breathe. When you are ready, raise your face and chest off the ground by pressing into the floor with your hands, arching your backing and gently bringing your relaxed gaze slightly up toward the ceiling. Hold for several deep breaths. Exhale and slowly lower yourself back onto the floor.

Upward Facing Dog Pose: This starts like the cobra pose, but unlike the former, in the upward facing dog pose lift your pelvis, knees, and quads off the ground an inch or so, by pressing into the floor with your hands and the tops of your feet.

If you find these poses helpful, you may want to consider finding a yoga class at your local gym or practicing at home with instructional videos on YouTube. Or, if you really like the feeling of yoga but the movement isn't for you, you may want to consider meditation. Meditation is a practice in which people "fall awake," and many meditators report feeling a renewed experience of alertness. You can meditate using the resources in Tip 4.

USE YOUR BODY CLOCK TO PLAN ACTIVITIES REQUIRING ALERTNESS

When you learned about your body clock in the Tip 2 chapter, you learned that you have a chronotype (that is, an ideal window for when you should sleep) that ranges from an extreme early bird to an extreme night owl. You also learned that most adults are somewhere in between an early bird and a night owl, but that there are developmental influences that can affect this. In particular, during puberty there is a shift toward being a night owl.

Chronotypes do not just determine your ideal sleep window; you can also use your chronotype information to determine your ideal alertness window, and schedule your most demanding activities during this high-alertness period. Early birds experience a burst of alertness in the morning hours and when they schedule activities during this window, this is their most productive time. Night owls tend to experience fairly low levels of alertness through the morning hours and experience a burst of alertness in the later afternoon to early evening hours. Unfortunately, when night owls start activities or projects or schoolwork or workouts at this time, some people criticize them for procrastinating. However, this is exactly when a night owl should be engaged in activities requiring alertness.

Explain to detractors that this is when you feel alert, and that you have difficulties with demanding activities earlier in the day. Unfortunately, school occurs during a night owl's lowest alertness. So if you are a night owl, try completing homework, studying, and other activities requiring alertness in the later afternoon and early evening, and rely on fatigue-management strategies such as HELM or yoga during the first half of the day when your alertness is low. It is important to disengage from alerting activities in the two hours before bed and to focus more on activities that are not goal-directed and are consistent with a wind-down from your day.

Summary

- Particular thoughts about fatigue can make it more likely that you will engage in fatigue-producing or sleep-interfering behaviors. It is important to challenge unhelpful thoughts about fatigue.

- Fatigue is caused by many things, including eating irregularly and unhealthily, caffeine withdrawal, boredom, underexertion, over-exertion, stress, anxiety, depressed mood, dehydration, sub-stances such as alcohol, medical conditions, medications, an irregular schedule for getting into and out of bed, and lingering in bed in the morning.

- There is a normal temporary dip in energy after lunch. Making a pre-sleep and pro-energy plan for the dip will lessen its impact.

- Fatigue is managed effectively with movement and activity, as well as with hydration, good nutrition, and light exposure.

Your Plan for the Week

☐ Challenge unhelpful thinking about fatigue.

☐ Use healthy coping strategies during the post-lunch dip: go for a walk, exercise, socialize, take a break, or do something fun.

☐ Reduce "jet lag without travel" fatigue symptoms by trying to go to bed at the same time, and trying to get up around the same time each morning.

☐ Get out of bed as quickly as possible after you wake up. Lingering in bed increases fatigue. Consider a good stretch or mountain pose to get things started.

☐ Experiment with activity, exercise, yoga, or meditation as healthy ways to manage or prevent fatigue.

☐ Stay hydrated, eat three healthy meals at regular times, and decrease your consumption of caffeinated products or other fatigue-producing substances.

☐ Work with your chronotype: shift tasks requiring alertness to the time of day in which you feel most alert.

Manage Substances That Rob You of Deep Sleep

Some people use substances to achieve specific feelings. For example, you may drink coffee or an energy drink when you want to feel more alert and energetic, or less fatigued. However, even though some substances may help you feel energetic, they can make you feel even more tired later and can interfere with your sleep. Even substances that make you feel relaxed or calm can cause problematic sleep disturbances, resulting in feeling even *more* tired the next day. Learning about substances that might be interfering with your sleep, and making a plan to stop or decrease your use of these substances, will help you sleep better.

USE YOUR SLEEP TRACKER TO PINPOINT PROBLEMS WITH SLEEP-INTERFERING SUBSTANCES

On your Sleep Tracker or using the DOZe app, did you answer "yes" to using sleep-interfering products? If so, it is probably better to track the amount and timing of these substances (particularly whether they occur within two hours of bedtime). If you are regularly consuming large amounts throughout the day, or consuming these products within an hour or two of bedtime, use this chapter and the Sleep Tracker or the DOZe app to track whether you meet your goals for reducing or quitting, and whether these changes result in improvements in the time it takes to fall asleep, the time awake during the night, or the efficiency of sleep.

The Case of Drew

Drew is a 16-year-old high school student with a problem falling asleep at night. His mother enforces a 10 p.m. lights-out policy, but Drew's body doesn't feel ready to sleep at that time. He lies in bed for several hours unable to sleep. In the past year, he has gone up to bed at 10 p.m. and turned off the light, but he games on his laptop for several hours before trying to sleep. He didn't feel tired after the several hours of gaming, so he began sneaking out to the second-story balcony of his house to smoke a joint. Drew says that he feels more relaxed after the joint. Nonetheless, he continued to have sleep problems and now his pattern is to smoke a joint around 11:30 p.m. or midnight and another just before trying to sleep around 1–2 a.m. Even though he continues to have sleep problems, Drew believes that his problems would be worse if he didn't smoke up.

The Case of Amy

Amy is a 15-year-old honor roll student with high grades, many friends, and many activities outside school, including a part-time job. Amy admits that she drinks a lot of caffeine over the course of the day, in part because she and her friends like to hang out at a coffee shop, but also to manage feeling tired. She has had trouble falling asleep since starting high school. Amy drinks energy drinks, diet sodas, and iced coffee drinks throughout the day and into the night. She denies that it has any effect on her sleep and believes she would not be able to function on less caffeine.

We will check in on Amy and Drew throughout this chapter. The use of hard substances like MDMA, heroin, and cocaine tends to be rare in teens, but there are other substances that are more common that can affect sleep in ways that you may not have considered. In this chapter, let's follow the two teens described above, who have a pattern of use that is more typical, and see how their substance use may be affecting their sleep problems. Then we'll look into some tactics to help change this use.

IDENTIFY SUBSTANCES THAT INTERFERE WITH DEEP SLEEP OR MAKE YOU TIRED

Caffeine. Caffeine is present in coffee, some teas (for example, black, green), soft drinks (for example, Pepsi, Coke, Dr. Pepper, Mountain Dew), energy drinks (for example, Red Bull, Monster Energy, 5-Hour Energy), chocolate, caffeine pills, and certain types of ice cream (for example, chocolate- or coffee-flavored).

Caffeine-based products like coffee may provide you with a welcome pick-me-up in the mornings or at times when energy is low (for example, when staying up late to study for a test). Although a cup or two of a caffeinated beverage may not be overly problematic for your sleep, heavy use may be causing some sleep interference. When taken late in the day or in the evening, it can really disrupt your sleep. Another thing to remember is that caffeine sometimes hides in places we wouldn't expect to find it, such as in your favorite chocolate bar or in your after-dinner bowl of ice cream. Check out the list above to see if you have been consuming caffeine without knowing it.

Caffeine has a long "half-life," which may sound familiar from chemistry class. This basically means that after using caffeine, the body has to process it and break it down, and this process takes a long time—sometimes many hours. While it may be obvious that drinking an energy drink at 10 p.m. will likely cause you some sleep problems, it might come as a surprise that having a cup of coffee in the early afternoon—even as early as 3 p.m.—can also result in sleep disturbances that night. This is because the caffeine might not yet be broken down and might still be circulating through the body many hours later. How sensitive a person is to caffeine varies widely, but people having sleep problems are generally advised to avoid caffeine use after 3 p.m. and not to drink more than half an energy drink (the equivalent of three cups of coffee) per day. As you can see in Amy's Substance Use Monitoring (which you can download at http://www.newharbinger.com/44383), she consumes much more than that, and some of it later in the day. You can use that same form to monitor your own substance use.

Nicotine. Nicotine is present in cigarettes, e-cigarettes, dip, chew, hookah, cigars, and pipes.

Nicotine is most commonly used in the form of cigarettes, but it is also found in other forms of tobacco like hookah and chewing tobacco, and even in e-cigarettes. Like caffeine, nicotine is a stimulant—among other things, it causes adrenaline to be released in your body and your heart rate and breathing rate to increase. So you may not be surprised to learn that using nicotine makes it harder to fall asleep and makes your sleep shorter. Nicotine also interferes with REM sleep, so that you might experience weirder dreams. In addition, inhaling smoke (whether it includes nicotine or not) increases the likelihood that you will become a snorer. Snoring is not only rather embarrassing, but it also reduces your overall sleep quality. Cigarette smoking has also been found to increase the likelihood of developing certain severe sleep disorders, and many smokers experience sleep difficulties (such as problems falling or staying asleep and feeling sleepy during the day) and use more caffeine during the day as a result. This is in addition to your risk of early death from cancers and so on, and the economic and social costs to engaging in a socially undesirable behavior.

If you use nicotine, it should always be on your list to stop, but if you have sleep problems and are using, that is an added important reason to prioritize quitting. That said, quitting is not easy and there is often an initial worsening of your sleep problem during quitting, so it is important to use as many resources as you can to help you manage. See the "Suggested Readings and Resources" list at www .newharbinger.com/44383.

Cannabis. Cannabis is variously known as weed, pot, hash, hashish, marijuana, bhang, grass, or hemp. At this time, less is known about the various forms of cannabis used for medical purposes. We are talking here about the more commonly used forms of "recreational" marijuana.

An important tool for changing substance-use patterns is to be fully aware of any possible downsides and dangers. In the case of marijuana, because it has been used in various forms in medical treatments and there is a growing pattern of decriminalization for adults, many people believe that marijuana is harmless and even helpful. You should know the facts, though.

First of all, it is important to remember that teen use of marijuana is still illegal everywhere, so its use can cause serious legal troubles.

It can also have significant health effects. Although teens may use cannabis products to feel relaxed, using marijuana before bed can actually disrupt your sleep over the whole night. The main reason for this is that while your body is eliminating the marijuana from your body, REM sleep is displaced temporarily. Later in your sleep cycle, REM sleep appears more intensely and longer—causing sleep to be light and broken, and perhaps increasing the likelihood of strange or disturbing dreams and sweating. Moreover, when you use marijuana, your body does not spend enough time in deep sleep. As you have learned already, deep, slow-wave sleep is important for helping us feel rested and refreshed during the day. Deep sleep is also extremely important for us because it is the part of sleep that produces hormones and chemicals that help our bodies and brains grow, learn, and heal. Long-term use of marijuana (nightly use for one month or more) can result in serious decreases in your ability to produce deep sleep.

There are lots of other reasons for teens not to use marijuana. Marijuana has a variety of negative effects on the teenage brain that can be long lasting, even into the twenties. These cognitive effects include problems with concentration, slower mental reactions, poor coordination, poor short-term memory, and slower time to react physically. These types of effects can have a negative impact on you at school, or at your part-time job, in sports, and while driving. Cannabis users may also suffer from effects like poor judgment, strange thoughts (even hallucinations), a distorted sense of time, and paranoia. And the effects may be variable: sometimes you will feel alert after cannabis and sometimes you will feel sleepy. Some teens use this drug to manage anxiety or depression, but it often actually makes these conditions worse. If you smoke or vape marijuana, there can be more tar and cancer-producing agents than even in cigarettes, which is linked to a risk of cancer or lung disease. Another concern is that, since it is illegal, buying marijuana from a drug dealer puts you in contact with someone who may encourage the use of other drugs, which can get you involved with increasingly more dangerous substances.

Remember Drew? In addition to understanding that his current pattern of use is interfering with his ability to produce deep sleep and that it makes his sleep less restorative, there are a number of other factors for Drew to consider. First, he continues to have sleep problems with the marijuana use. Moreover, he has increased his marijuana use and it has not had a positive effect on his sleep. It's time for Drew to consider that marijuana is not helpful and that there may be other factors to consider. We will check in with Drew later in the chapter.

Alcohol. Alcohol is present in beer, wine, liquor, and liqueurs.

Another substance that is illegal for teens is alcohol. Sometimes teens use alcohol as a way of trying to avoid negative emotions (such as worry, sadness, or social anxiety). You may find that it initially makes you feel more relaxed, but you will soon also find that you need more alcohol to achieve that same feeling. This means that you will be drinking more and more. This is both illegal and expensive, and it can have a variety of other negative effects, such as vomiting, feeling too sick the next day for school or for your part-time job, impairing your ability to drive, leaving you vulnerable to something bad happening to you if you pass out, or even possible death (for example, vomiting and subsequently choking while passed out). Although people say that alcohol makes them feel drowsy and helps them fall asleep more quickly, the effectiveness of alcohol quickly fades as it takes more and more alcohol to achieve the same sedating effect. Moreover, the overall impact of alcohol on sleep is not good. If you go to bed with alcohol in your system, the overall *quality* of your sleep will be very poor. Some people will notice that they wake up more frequently or feel as though they never get into a "deep" sleep. Others might feel that they slept through the night but wake up in the morning feeling unrested and exhausted. Any amount of alcohol taken before bed (even just one drink) can cause disruptions in your sleep, especially in the second half of the night.

Opioids. Opioids include OxyContin, Percocet, oxycodone, codeine, fentanyl, Vicodin, hydrocodone opiates, methadone, and morphine.

Opioids are prescribed by doctors for treatment of chronic medical conditions. If this is the case for you, be sure to discuss any questions you have about your medications before making any changes. However, some teens use narcotics even though they have not been prescribed by a medical professional. Teens take narcotic medications for many reasons, such as to feel relaxed or to reduce feelings of pain. Depending on the type of narcotic taken, the effects on sleep can vary, but narcotic use often results in some form of sleep difficulty—especially if narcotics are taken regularly or over a long period of time. Using narcotics increases the time you will spend awake in the middle of the night, may make it more difficult to fall asleep at night, and also changes your sleep pattern over the course of the night. In addition, narcotic use makes the *quality* of your sleep worse. The main reason is that your body doesn't spend enough time in an important stage of sleep—deep sleep, or slow-wave sleep—that helps you feel rested and refreshed during the day. Opioids can make you feel sleepy, confused, and nauseated. But beyond sleep, these medications have turned deadly for many people. They can cause death due to overdose, even from just one use. They are highly addictive and can lead to taking other harmful drugs too. It is important to seek help when attempting to reduce or quit.

Other Illegal Drugs. The substances below are illegal, which has potential implications for your record and even your freedom. They are bad for your health and can cause an early death. They are also sleep-interfering in various ways. They tend to interfere with your sleep cycles, which can result in changes to REM sleep (interfering with learning and memory) and deep sleep (important for helping you feel rested and refreshed during the day, as well as for growth and tissue restoration or healing). Some medications create difficulties falling asleep and some cause you to fall asleep during the day.

Almost all interfere with the quality of sleep, making it light and fitful.

- *Cocaine, Crack Cocaine* (coke, crack, blow, rock, yeyo, bumps): Cocaine is a stimulant drug that causes increased wakefulness, meaning that falling asleep and staying asleep are quite difficult after using it. Cocaine interferes with REM sleep, so you feel like you had very poor quality sleep and will feel fatigued the next day. Also, once the immediate effects of cocaine wear off, people will often go into cocaine withdrawal. Withdrawal from cocaine causes unpleasant dreams and additional sleep disturbances for many people.

- *MDMA* (m, ecstasy, e, molly): MDMA causes disturbed sleep, in part because of its alerting properties. Using MDMA frequently or in high doses is not only dangerous to your general health but also causes long-term sleep disturbances and changes the structure of your sleep and the way that your body cycles through the different stages of sleep. This is a huge problem because our bodies are designed to cycle through these stages in a certain pattern, and messing with that pattern leads to long-term, even lifelong, sleep difficulties.

- *Heroin* (tar, china, dope, smack, junk): Heroin is extremely addictive, and extremely dangerous to your overall health and development. Heroin has an interfering effect on sleep, causing poor quality sleep and shortened sleep, and it changes the way your body cycles through the different stages of sleep.

- *Hallucinogens* (acid, tabs, LSD): LSD or acid causes sleep difficulties such as waking up more frequently during the night and increased body movements while sleeping. After using LSD, you will also have a poorer *quality* sleep. While you might expect your sleep to be disturbed the night after using LSD, these sleep disturbances can actually continue to be a problem many weeks after LSD use, so it is important to consider stopping using LSD altogether.

- *Amphetamines* (speed, crank, upper, tweek): Sometimes people use amphetamines or speed to increase their energy level. People who use amphetamines are not particularly surprised to learn that it disrupts their sleep. Amphetamines are stimulants that cause increased wakefulness, meaning that falling asleep and staying asleep are quite difficult after using them. After using amphetamines, you will spend less time in REM sleep, resulting in a poorer overall sleep quality and feelings of fatigue the next day.

MAKE A SUCCESSFUL PLAN FOR REDUCING SUBSTANCES THAT ROB YOU OF SLEEP

Sometimes it is difficult to make a change because you are not sure if you want to make the change. Write down the reasons why you do not want to make the change, and then write down all the reasons why you do want to make the change. Spend some time on this list. What are all the things you lose by not making the change? What are all the things you gain by making the change? When we see these lists side by side, we often move closer to considering a change.

"I hate how I feel the next day."

"I want to sleep better."

"I am worried about my health if I keep taking it."

"It costs so much money."

"I was so scared when I was pulled over for speeding that I was going to be arrested for possession. I've got to get this problem under control."

Seeing all the negatives of taking the substance and what you will gain by making the change may help you commit to quitting. See the downloadable form Pros and Cons of Using Something That Hurts Sleep (http://www.newharbinger.com/44383), which includes Amy's completed form so that you can see how she made the decision to reduce her caffeine consumption.

MAKE A BEHAVIORAL PLAN FOR REDUCING SUBSTANCES

The most successful behavior change occurs when a plan is:

1. *Realistic:* If you are using a substance nightly, it is probably unrealistic to go cold turkey and stop it altogether. A goal in which you decrease by a set amount, or eliminate a particular number of days per week, is often a better starting point.

Amy decides that she is going to start decreasing her caffeine use by substituting noncaffeinated beverages.

2. *Specific:* A goal in which you decrease by a specific (written-down) amount, or in which you eliminate a particular number of days per week, makes it easier to stick to your plan. As you can see on Amy's Substance Monitoring form (which you can view or download at http://www.new harbinger.com/44383), she drank an average of six caffeinated drinks per day. She is already drinking less on weekends, so she figures that it would be manageable to decrease her use on weekdays to match. She decides that she will drink a maximum of three caffeinated drinks per day and will replace all other drinks with a decaf or noncaffeinated option. None of the three caffeinated drinks will be consumed later than 1 p.m.

3. *Measureable:* Track your results and see if your goal was realistic or if you need more help in place to achieve your goal. We have included a tracking form just like Amy's (which you can download at http://www.newharbinger. com/44383) for you to track your progress.

If you make a plan, it is important that you write it down. The plan should have many steps in it. It should include a plan if you relapse—this is a normal part of the process. You should look at your plan every day, as you may forget some parts of the plan, and this allows you to recommit to the plan every day. Commit each day and you will be less likely to stray.

Don't Go It Alone

Making changes is best done with lots of help. When you have people around, they can help you remain accountable. They also can provide encouragement and may have resources to share (for example, friends can provide support and encouragement, counselors can give tips and support, family doctors can provide a medical plan).

Be Kind to Yourself When You Forget

Forgive yourself and get right back into your plan. Setbacks are normal. The important thing is not to let them become permanent setbacks. Criticizing yourself, or telling yourself that now that you have relapsed you might as well smoke the whole pack, will create a greater setback and make it harder to get back on track.

USE OTHER STRATEGIES TO REPLACE THE SUBSTANCE

Remember Drew? He continues to have sleep problems even though he has increased his marijuana use. It's time for him to realize that marijuana is not helpful and that there are other factors to consider. For example, could his pattern of gaming contribute to staying up later? He could test this in an experiment. He could try a week in which he engages in something like reading or listening to music and compare his sleep to a week in which he is using active gaming. It is possible that Drew needs even more strategies as a wind-down, perhaps some anxiety-management techniques like mindfulness or meditation. Engaging in a healthier relaxation strategy may help him fall asleep earlier. It may also make sense for Drew and his mother to negotiate a later bedtime, so that he is not spending so much time in his bed awake when there is no chance of falling asleep. Engaging in a wind-down earlier outside of the bedroom, using anxiety-management strategies, and trying some of the night owl strategies in Tip 2, Drew now has a plan that allows him to avoid the negative effects of marijuana and to stop a strategy that isn't working.

GET PROFESSIONAL HELP

There are many options to help you decrease or stop substances that are harmful, including talking to your family doctor and using the "Suggested Readings and Resources" list at http://www.new harbinger.com/44383 for relevant websites, apps, and support. You have so much to gain by decreasing or stopping your use of the substances covered in this chapter, but it is important to have some support. Doctors are helpful for keeping you safe as you decrease or stop, and they can provide medications or other means to make it easier. A support group can help you commit to a change once it has occurred. Ongoing counseling can help with managing stress, as stress can increase urges and make it more difficult to commit to your plan. Trusted friends and family can be much-needed cheerleaders for your accomplishments and can also hold you accountable and get you back on track during slips. The more people who can provide information, help, and support, the more likely it is that you will be successful.

Summary

- Substances, even if taken specifically to make you feel sleepy enough to fall asleep, tend to end up being sleep-disruptive.

- Substances, even if taken specifically to make you feel more energetic, tend to end up being sleep-disruptive.

- In addition to being sleep-disruptive, some of the substances covered in this chapter are illegal, extremely unhealthy, and potentially deadly.

- You are strongly encouraged to set a goal for this week, to either reduce or stop taking sleep-interfering substances during this week.

Your Plan for the Week

☐ Make a list of all the reasons why it would be a good or bad idea to quit.

☐ Make your goal for reducing or quitting realistic, specific, and measureable, and track your results.

☐ If you are planning on reducing or stopping a substance altogether this week, you should make a list of the resources you will use. A good place to start is your family doctor.

Think Like a Good Sleeper

The way that you think about sleep is important. Good sleepers have beliefs about sleep that tend to protect them during times of sleep disruption. They have confidence that any problems with their sleep will pass, and they trust their body to make up for sleep loss naturally. Good sleepers do not spend a lot of time trying to control their sleep or their sleep environment. They remove things that can get in the way of good sleep, such as noise (for example, turning off phone notifications) or light (for example, ensuring that screens are off when they are in bed), but do not spend a ton of effort trying to control their sleep environment (for example, they don't buy black-out blinds, sleep masks, herbal supplements, white noise machines, special mattresses or pillows, or apps to try to make themselves fall sleep). They understand that regular daytime activity, a regular wind-down period before bed, and a somewhat regular sleep schedule are probably all they need to do to allow their body to produce sleep naturally. If good sleepers have a bad night, they assume the next night will be okay.

In other words, good sleepers *get* that they need sleep and they attempt to have a regular schedule, enough daytime activity, and enough time (and not much more) to sleep at night. *How* you think determines *what* you do (that is, what your sleep behaviors will be), so how you think is very important in how you subsequently sleep. This chapter will teach you to discover if you think like a poor sleeper, and if you do, how you can change your thinking about sleep to something more helpful. Managing thoughts that get in the way of good sleep (1) allows you to make different choices about sleep behaviors, (2) makes you feel less anxious about sleep, and, as a result, (3) can pave the way to good sleep.

DISCOVER IF YOU THINK LIKE A POOR SLEEPER

Good and poor sleepers tend to differ in their beliefs about sleep. Look at the beliefs below to determine if you tend to identify more with good sleeper or poor sleeper thoughts.

1. Do you think in extreme, all-or-nothing terms?

Poor sleeper belief: I need 8 hours of sleep or I won't be able to function during the day.

OR

Good sleeper belief: I feel at my best when I get about 8 hours of sleep, but I can still function during the day.

Relative to good sleepers, poor sleepers overestimate the effects of poor sleep on how they will function the next day. Poor sleepers tend to see functioning in black-or-white terms, rather than considering the in-between grays. In other words, the only two options are the extremes: "I am functionally at my best" or "I am not functioning at all." In reality, there is no such thing as not functioning. There is a wide range for how well you are functioning, and a good sleeper is more likely to think some version of: "I am not at my best today, but I'm okay." Good sleepers notice that sometimes they feel good and perform well during the day, even with poor sleep, and they can sometimes feel sleepy and struggle even when they had a good sleep.

2. Do you tend to think about the worst-case scenario, or to assume the worst?

Poor sleeper belief: My sleep system is broken and I'll never be able to sleep well again.

OR

Good sleeper belief: I'm annoyed that I'm having trouble sleeping, but it will correct itself soon.

Relative to good sleepers, poor sleepers tend to worry that poor sleep is a sign of a very serious medical problem with their sleep system. Besides being untrue (sleep systems do not "break"), believing the worst (that is, that your sleep system has failed) fuels further worry, and makes it difficult to sleep. This becomes a vicious worry cycle that becomes difficult to turn off. Good sleepers consider other possibilities to explain their current sleep difficulty, such as stress or their sleep habits, and assume that things will get better.

3. Are you prone to overestimations or misattributions when under stress?

Poor sleeper belief: If I feel exhausted during the day, it must be because I slept poorly last night.

OR

Good sleeper belief: If I feel exhausted during the day, it could be due to any number of things, like that I am bored, or that I have eaten unhealthy food, or that I need to drink some water.

Relative to good sleepers, poor sleepers tend to assume that any experiences of low mood or fatigue are always due to poor sleep. Fatigue is due to so many factors and if you think it is solely your sleep, you will feel helpless to do things that manage fatigue.

4. Do you strongly believe that you need to engage in a particular ritual in order to sleep?

Poor sleeper belief: I can't sleep without a TV on.

OR

Good sleeper belief: I'm sure I'll fall asleep no matter what.

Your body will produce sleep eventually if you have been sufficiently active, your schedule is regular, and you have allowed yourself some time to wind down. If you believe there is something you need to do, then if you have a poor night's sleep, you will become even more anxious, thinking your ritual no longer works, instead of realizing that it never worked as well as you thought it did. After all, if television or any other ritual had magical sleep properties, you would not be reading this book. What happens if the power goes out, or you have to sleep somewhere without a television? This will generate considerable anxiety and lead to a self-fulfilling prophesy in which you will not sleep well, and that will strengthen your belief that televisions are needed to sleep. (Actually, televisions left on during the night disrupt sleep, so this belief is particularly unhelpful.)

If you tended to identify with the thoughts of a poor sleeper, that may be a factor in your sleep problem.

The Case of Nadia

Nadia was a senior, focused on trying to get A's on her upcoming report card. She had high standards for herself and worked very hard. This strategy worked well for her. She had great grades and was the captain of the volleyball team and the top volleyball player in her school district. But Nadia had trouble falling asleep at night and felt tired during the day. Nadia believed that a key to her success in school was getting at least eight hours of sleep every night. She believed that if she wasn't asleep within five minutes then she would "never" get to sleep and her "whole day would be ruined." She believed that if she "put her mind to it," she could will herself out of her sleep problem. After all, the strategy of putting all her focus and effort into a problem worked in every other aspect of her life very well, so why not do the same for sleep? She spent lots of time on the Internet reading sleep blogs and searching for solutions. She talked every day to her friends about how poorly she slept the night before, how tired she felt during the day, and what new sleep tips or products she read

*about. She tried everything. Every night she took melatonin she
bought at a health food store. She worried that she had some sort
of virus that was interfering with her melatonin production
(because she had read that melatonin helped you fall asleep). She
insisted that her parents set the thermostat at a particular
temperature, she wore a sleep mask, and she listened to sounds
of the ocean on her phone. Nothing worked, and Nadia was
frustrated and anxious about her situation. She was concerned
that the sleep problem was going to negatively affect her grades
and ruin her chances of getting into a good college.*

Do you think Nadia thinks like a good sleeper or a poor sleeper?
Nadia thinks in extreme, all-or-nothing terms. She believes her
whole day is ruined when she has a poor night, rather than considering she might not feel that bad, or that if she does feel bad, there are
things she can do to cope with the symptoms of sleep loss. She is
prone to thinking about the worst-case scenario. For example, she
thinks she has a melatonin problem in her body and believes that
her sleep problem is going to undermine her efforts in getting into a
good college. There is no evidence that insomnia is caused by a
chemical imbalance or a melatonin problem, so to jump to that con-
clusion is catastrophizing. Additionally, assuming that poor sleep
will automatically lead to a cascade of events that will result in her
getting into a "bad" college is likely an exaggeration. She is also
prone to overestimating the effect of her sleep problem on how she
feels during the day. She has not considered that the pressure she
puts on herself to achieve at a high level and her unrealistic sleep
standards could be causing anxiety and fatigue during the day.

Nadia also believes in engaging in rituals to sleep, even though they don't work that well (melatonin, a particular temperature, masks, ocean sounds, and so on). Engaging in those rituals means that she has little confidence in her body's ability to produce sleep naturally. If she were to learn how her body works and work in cooperation with her body, she would be able to sleep well and it would help rebuild her sleep confidence.

But is changing Nadia's thoughts the key to helping her sleep better? Let's follow Nadia throughout the chapter.

CONNECT THOUGHTS TO THEIR MOST LIKELY CONSEQUENCE

Having all-or-nothing, worst-case scenario, or misattribution beliefs can make the sleep problem worse. Connecting these thoughts to their consequences can increase your motivation to do something to challenge these thoughts when they arise. Let's revisit Nadia and compare her to her friend, Devania. Both Devania and Nadia struggle all night long to sleep.

Devania thinks, "That sucked, but I'll be okay."

Nadia thinks, "That sucked. I'm never going to be able to make it through the day."

Both thoughts acknowledge that the sleeplessness was a negative experience, which is important to note. The solution isn't just to "think positive," because this ignores the fact that it does feel unpleasant to have a sleep problem. But there is a key difference between the two thoughts. Devania's thought makes a positive prediction and Nadia's thought makes a negative prediction for the rest of the day. There is nothing wrong with either thought, but the two thoughts will probably have different outcomes.

The good news is that you can make changes to the way you think in the moment, and it can change how you feel and what you do. It is powerful to understand that change in one area affects the others. For example, if you wake up to your alarm feeling groggy and have the thought, "If I am tired, it must mean I should stay in bed and sleep in," this thought will lead you to sleep in, having a negative impact on your body clock, your energy level, and your deep sleep the next night. If you challenge this thought and instead think, "I can shake off this feeling more quickly if I get up. If I sleep in, I might be late for class, feel jet-lagged during the day, and be less able to get deep sleep tonight," it would likely lead to a more helpful coping behavior.

CHANGE THOUGHTS THAT GET IN THE WAY OF CHANGE

Some beliefs about sleep get in the way of making the changes necessary to sleep better. When you find yourself upset, or when your sleep problems are particularly challenging:

1. STOP.

2. Breathe.

3. Check your thoughts. Write down the thoughts you are having. If there is one thought that seems more emotionally charged than the other thoughts, focus on that particular

thought. Question the thought to determine if the thought you are having in this situation is making the situation better or worse. For example, Nadia had the thought, "I am going to do poorly in school today," in response to having a poor night's sleep. This thought made her very anxious and focused on looking for proof that she was not functioning as well as she wanted, which made her even more anxious. So now, in addition to having a poor night's sleep, her energy is taken up looking for proof, rather than focusing on her schoolwork, and anxiety is taking resources away from focusing on her schoolwork as well. Was this thought helpful for Nadia? The answer is no. There are questions she could ask herself to consider thoughts that are more helpful, and to consider thoughts that do not lead to more problems. Not so sure you know how to do this? Read the next section, "Questions That Tip You Off That the Thought Is Unhelpful."

4. Test your thought. Do an experiment to test if the thought is actually true or helpful. For example, Nadia believed that if she had a poor night's sleep, she should cancel hanging out with friends so that she could work even harder. This meant that she never took a break and had no stress relief for that day. Is it possible that you need breaks to perform well? Nadia could test whether canceling is more helpful by keeping track of her mood, fatigue, and sleep during a week in which she did not allow herself breaks. She could then spend a week allowing herself her regular breaks to test whether it is more helpful not to deprive herself. You can

read more about how to test your thoughts in the "Test Your Thoughts" section below.

QUESTIONS THAT TIP YOU OFF THAT THE THOUGHT IS UNHELPFUL

Above, you were asked to stop, breathe, and check your thoughts by writing them down. Once you have written your thought down, here are some questions to ask yourself to see if the thought you are having is causing problems for you.

Is this thought true 100% of the time? If you believe that because you are having the thought, somehow it must be true, it may lead you to more distress and to coping behaviors that are unhelpful. Think about times when the thought is *not* true. For example, "I can't go to school if I have poor sleep." This can't be true 100% of the time, right? Haven't you gone to school when you have slept poorly? Believing the thought that you *cannot* go to school will make it more likely you will not go to school. Not going to school can create academic problems by causing you to get behind at school, and absences can get you in trouble. This can also create conflict with your parents. It also makes you feel less confident about whether you can cope with sleep loss. This one little thought can have several negative effects, so it is something that is unhelpful and worth challenging. If you are able to, consider another thought: "I don't feel like going to school when I have poor sleep, but if I do, it will be more helpful for my sleep, my schoolwork, and my sleep confidence than if I skip."

Does this thought lead you to feel less confident about your sleep, and about your ability to cope? If you believe that you cannot go to school whenever you have a poor night's sleep, it suggests that you have very little confidence in your ability to cope. By not going to school, you are not able to see yourself challenging the belief that you cannot be at school, so the belief will persist. If you were to go to school and observe yourself coping, it would strengthen the belief in yourself that you can cope with problems. In other words, if you go to school, it actively challenges the thought that you are a victim of your sleep problem and that there is nothing you can do about it. By going to school, you also have not added the problems associated with skipping school. A shift in this thought allows you to avoid the problems associated with skipping school and protects your confidence in yourself as someone who can cope well.

Does this thought lead you to engage in behaviors that would be helpful or sleep-interfering? A thought about skipping school because of a poor night is more likely to lead to similar avoiding behaviors. Avoiding activities when you sleep poorly removes a regular activity from your schedule, so there will be less regular cues for your body clock, which means more "jet lag without travel" symptoms (for example, fatigue and mood problems). Avoiding activities also results in less deep sleep drive. Avoidance of school can have a host of other negative consequences, including increased anxiety about being able to catch up on missed work. So, avoidance leads to worsened sleep, and sometimes also to increased anxiety.

What would you say to someone you loved who was in the same situation? It is often easier to have compassionate and encouraging things to say to someone else. But why are you the big exception? What makes you so special that you don't need and deserve encouragement and compassion? The answer is that you too need encouragement. So what would you say to someone else you cared about? "I'd probably tell them that they have to go to school sometime. They can't just drop out of school. I'd probably tell them to take care of themselves as best they could to get through the school day." Do you see how this new thought makes it more likely that you would go to school and have a better day? Just by considering alternative thoughts, you can see improvements in your mood immediately and it makes it more likely that you will act in a way that will support healthy coping. Use the Question Your Thoughts worksheet (which you can download at http://www.newharbinger.com/44383) to help you work through unhelpful thinking.

TEST YOUR THOUGHTS

Sometimes we are overly impressed with our own thoughts. It is as if the very fact that you have the thought makes it true. Really? Let's see if that's so. One thought that many poor sleepers have is that when you have a sleep problem, you should conserve your energy and rest. But you have learned that increased rest decreases the drive for deep sleep and actually increases fatigue.

If you are unsure whether you believe this new information, how would you test this out? In a good experiment, it should be clear exactly what thought or belief you are testing, and also what alternative thought might be true. In this case, you are testing whether conserving energy actually makes you feel less tired; the other possibility is that it makes you more tired and that you need to expend a little energy to get energy and to sleep well. Carry out experiments using the downloadable Test Your Thoughts form (which you can download at http://www.newharbinger.com/44383) to test if your thoughts are actually true or helpful. It is helpful for people actually to experience that they have less fatigue when they use some energy. Using the Sleep Tracker can also help confirm this.

SHIFTING FOCUS AWAY FROM SLEEP PREOCCUPATION

You need to sleep to live, not live to sleep. Remember when Nadia spent considerable time on the Internet learning about insomnia tips and talked all day with her friends about her sleep problem? If all you can think about is sleep, you are likely to continue having a sleep problem. If you are having a sleep problem, it is difficult to think about anything else. Telling yourself, "Do *not* think about sleep," is easier said than done. Below are some strategies that have been shown to be more helpful than trying to stop certain thoughts.

Distraction. Many people with sleep problems tell themselves, "Don't think about [*insert whatever you don't want to think about here*]." But *not* thinking about something is really still thinking about some aspect of the thing you don't want to think about. In other words, it doesn't work to try hard not to think about something. If I told you: *Do NOT think of chocolate cake fresh out of the oven. Do not think of the smell. Do not picture the steam rising off of it. Do not imagine how it tastes in your mouth.* How successful would that be? Instead of forcing yourself *not* to think of something, *do* something active. Watch, listen, or read something engaging. Socialize. Go for a walk. Switch things around to shake up the situation that led to the thought in the first place. I find that teens are more likely to have a distressing recurrent thought when they are disengaged from their environment, and especially when they are not particularly active.

Acceptance. Instead of distracting or activating or challenging your thoughts, another way to experience that your thoughts aren't facts is to simply observe them. The next time you are in a situation in which you are having distressing thoughts, shift your attention to writing out the words, or simply imagine the words of the thought written on signs carried in a parade. See the words of the thought on the sign and watch it march out of view. If another thought emerges, write that down on the sign and watch it march away. This exercise teaches you to be more of an observer of your thoughts.

If I told you that Nadia has the thought that she can't cope with sleep loss, Nadia's thought doesn't carry an emotional charge for you and her thought would disappear from your mind fairly quickly, because you don't even know Nadia. In other words, the idea does not take over your attention because Nadia's thoughts are not as relevant to you. This means that you are capable of distancing yourself from other people's thoughts. But when a thought relates to you,

you may become stuck on the personal implications of the thought. However, your thought is no different than Nadia's, and doing this exercise will help you get off a negative thought cycle.

WHEN SELF-CRITICAL THOUGHTS GET IN THE WAY OF MAKING CHANGES

Some people say that it is helpful to be demanding of themselves, as it helps them achieve. This was a key strategy for Nadia, and it worked to help her achieve A's in school and be one of the best volleyball players. But although this may be helpful in some areas of your life, your inner voice can also switch into being unhelpful without your being aware of it. For example, if your inner voice is critical, harsh, or demanding, this can leave you feeling discouraged and feeling negatively about yourself. Worse still, some people find these self-critical statements upsetting but do not challenge them because they believe these thoughts must be true, because the thoughts sound so compelling. These types of thoughts are not peaceful, and they interfere with sleep. Moreover, they can undermine your attempts at behavior change.

If you notice that you are having trouble getting out of bed and you criticize yourself harshly, your mood will get worse and you will feel less motivated. Don't believe me? If your best friend was training for a marathon and was having trouble getting past 10 kilometers, what would be most helpful for them to hear?

"You're worthless. You should give up. What's wrong with you that you can't get past 10 kilometers? You're being lazy."

OR

"You can do this. Maybe you can stay at this distance for another week to build up even more stamina, and you can try something new next week to add just one more kilometer."

Encouragement is important for pursuing goals. Nadia can remind herself of her goals and push herself to put in some extra practice on the volleyball court or make some extra study notes for a test, but she can do this much better with encouragement. ("You've got this. Just 15 minutes more on the treadmill…you can do it!") She can even schedule in some rewards for meeting goals. ("I'm going to get my favorite smoothie when I get this done!") What works for Nadia as encouraging self-talk or reward may not work for you. Start your own practice to encourage yourself and soften overly harsh self-defeating thoughts.

SHIFTING FOCUS TO SLEEP: YOU NEED TO SLEEP TO LIVE

Of course, if you *never* think about sleep and you are having trouble staying awake during the day, you may have the opposite problem as those with insomnia. In other words, instead of overfocusing on sleep, you may not be focusing on it enough. If you think you don't need sleep, this is a big problem, because you will suffer from daytime sleepiness and may fall asleep during classes, which can result in poor performance at school, or even accidents if you are driving. A positive relationship with sleep means prioritizing getting enough time in bed, having a healthy amount of activity during the day, having a good wind-down period, and avoiding sleep-interfering substances. Just as it is important to challenge beliefs about sleep being the most important thing in your life (overfocusing on sleep), it is as important to challenge beliefs about not needing sleep.

A STRONG BELIEF ABOUT NOT NEEDING SLEEP CAN BE A SIGN OF A DIFFERENT PROBLEM

If there are periods in which you feel like you do not need to sleep for days at a time, and you also experience any of the following symptoms, you should talk to your family doctor, as these can be signs of another problem:

- You are speaking more quickly than usual.

- Your thoughts are racing.

- You feel increased energy and may engage in a lot more physical activity than usual.

- Your mood is hyper-positive with an exaggerated optimism.

- Your mood is very irritable: you feel impatient and perhaps act aggressively toward others.

- Your behavior is impulsive: for example, you find yourself spending lots of money, getting into trouble with the law, making rash decisions, or engaging in dangerous driving.

- You have an unusually inflated sense of self-importance, or think that you are invincible.

Summary

- Having untrue thoughts about sleep can lead to undesirable results, such as distress or other negative moods, and to behaviors that make the situation worse in the long term.

- It is less about whether a belief is true and more about how strongly or inflexibly you believe something to be true, and whether this pattern is unhelpful.

- When thoughts are upsetting, you can more closely examine them by asking yourself critical questions to determine if they are unhelpful.

- In addition to challenging negative thoughts to lessen their impact, you can also try distraction or acceptance. This is particularly helpful if you find that you are preoccupied with sleep.

- If you believe that sleep is a waste of time or that you do not need it, this belief can similarly lead to serious problems.

Your Plan for the Week

What will be your plan for your thoughts this week? Think of the possible plans below and determine which ones you will test out.

☐ I discovered I think like a good sleeper, so I don't intend to make any plans for changing thoughts this week.

☐ I will keep track of my thoughts and challenge thoughts that lead to increased distress, anxiety, or frustration, using the Question Your Thoughts form (downloadable at http://www.newharbinger. com/44383).

☐ I will try distraction, challenging, and acceptance if I find myself being preoccupied with sleep.

☐ I will test out pervasive beliefs in an experiment.

☐ I will challenge unhelpful beliefs about not needing sleep.

Make a New Plan If Your Sleep Remains a Problem

There are several reasons why you may not get the results that you wanted in addressing your sleep problem. First, there are many things that can get in the way of making changes, so it is important to evaluate what changes have been made and what changes were not possible or proved too difficult. It is important to reflect back on what worked, what didn't, and where you may have been stuck, in order to determine an immediate plan, as well as a future plan, for your sleep. It is also important to consider whether you have sleep problems other than, or in addition to, your original sleep complaint that require further consultation with your doctor.

KEEP IT REAL—USE EVIDENCE TO EVALUATE YOUR RESULTS

The Sleep Tracker is essential to success in this book. Tailored sleep schedules are often the main solution to a sleep difficulty, and holding yourself accountable on a Sleep Tracker will not only allow you to see whether you are following your plan as closely as you think, but it will also allow you to see whether it is working. If completing the Tracker is the problem, there is a recommended free Sleep Tracker app called DOZe (Delivering Online zzz's) that will be helpful as an accompaniment to this book. As said above, the core of this treatment is completing a Tracker, so this is always the most likely culprit for not getting the results you want.

IS YOUR CURRENT SLEEP HEALTHY FOR YOUR AGE?

Look at your Tracker results over the last week or two and check to see whether your sleep is about average, compared to other young adults.

- Are you asleep about 85–90% of the time (remember this is your sleep efficiency, calculated in the Sleep Tracker chapter)?

- Do you fall asleep on average after 10 to 30 minutes in bed?

- Once asleep, for the remainder of your time in bed, do you spend less than 30 minutes awake?

- Do you sleep between 8 and 10 hours (or between 7 and 9 hours if you are over 18 years old)?

If you answered yes to a question, it means that you are healthy on that particular index. Are most of your indices healthy? If yes, it is important to consider whether you believe you have a sleep problem because of the way that you feel during the day. If this is the case, the sections in this chapter on "Experiencing Common

Difficulties with the Treatment" and "Is It Time to See a Sleep Specialist?" may be particularly useful. Additionally, if you did not read the chapter on fatigue (Tip 7) and the "Think Like a Good Sleeper" chapter (Tip 9), they may also be helpful.

ARE THERE ANY HABITS GETTING IN THE WAY OF SLEEP?

If your sleep is not what is considered healthy, look at the list of common habits that interfere with sleep and check off which ones apply to you. Avoiding these habits consistently is the key to success, so even if you are doing them only occasionally, you may want to consider whether goal setting around a habit would help.

- Do you spend too much time in bed *or* too little time in bed? A healthy time is 8.5–10.5 hours in bed (or 7.5–9.5 hours if you are over 18 years old).

- Do you linger in bed in the morning more than 30 minutes past the alarm, or past the regular rise time?

- Do you suffer from morning jet lag? That is, is there an hour or more in variability between your earliest and latest rise time within the week?

- Do you suffer from bedtime jet lag? In other words, is there an hour or more in variability between your earliest and latest time going to bed within the week?

- Is your bed a place where you do wakeful activities (instead of being reserved for sleep only)?

- Do you set aside time for yourself to unwind every night (that is, winding down at least an hour before bed, preferably not on a screen and preferably outside of the bedroom)?

- Do you nap for alleviating sleepiness (as opposed to for safety)?

- Are you sleepy? Remember that sleepiness is: (1) falling asleep on average in less than 10 minutes, (2) spending more than 90% of the time that you are in bed asleep, or (3) falling asleep involuntarily during the day.

- Do you use sleep-interfering substances (for example, juling/smoking/vaping, marijuana, excessive caffeine)?

MAKING A NEW PLAN

So you evaluated your sleep and sleep habits in the previous section and you can see that there remain some problems that could be the difference in getting the results you want. Do you want to make a new plan for targeting these problems? If so, it may help to go back to the relevant chapter to help you with setting a goal and troubleshooting. Writing goals down and tracking them on the Sleep Tracker is a tried-and-true way to help you achieve your goal and to assess and whether or not a particular strategy has been helpful. If you are not sure about setting a new goal because you previously set goals and weren't able to follow through, it may be that there are things in your way. If there are, read on, because there are some tips that may help.

BARRIERS TO FEELING BETTER

There are many reasons you may have had trouble achieving your goal. There are difficulties you can experience with the treatment strategies themselves that may need to be addressed before you can move forward with your goal. There may be a barrier unique to you that needs to be identified, and you may need to brainstorm a list of possible solutions. It may be that you simply need another person to help you achieve your goal. It may be that keeping the behavior we recommend that you change (for example, refraining from over-sleeping on a weekend) is more important to you than working on your sleep problem. Or it may be that you have another sleep disorder that needs further evaluation and treatment. We address each below.

EXPERIENCING COMMON DIFFICULTIES WITH THE TREATMENT

Feeling tired during the day: If you read Tip 7 about managing fatigue, you learned that fatigue and sleep are only loosely associated; in other words, people make the assumption that feeling poorly during the day is because of sleep, but you should consider that feeling tired may be due to something else. If you have not read Tip 7, it would be helpful to read it now, and implement strategies like HELM (hydrating, eating three regular healthy meals, light exposure, and moving). If you read it, made changes, and your sleep has improved but you still don't feel better during the day, there are also several explanations to consider.

Feeling sleepy during the day: If you read Tip 5, you learned about sleepiness and how it is different from fatigue. Sleepiness is the propensity to fall asleep quickly, and when it occurs during the day, it can be dangerous. When you are falling asleep too quickly at night, it implies that you need more of a sleep opportunity. You should use the advice in that chapter to alleviate sleepiness if you are experiencing it. Here were some of the strategies:

- Add half an hour to your time in bed during the week, and use the Sleep Tracker to determine if you get more sleep and feel better.

- Nap for safety when experiencing sleepiness. Napping is not typically needed or advised on the weekend, unless you are about to drive and feel sleepy. If you are about to drive and feel sleepy, take a nap first or find an alternative way to get to your destination.

- If sleepiness remains, it is important to talk about your sleepiness with your family doctor.

TROUBLESHOOT!

Knowing that something works for most people may not be enough to convince you to make the change. It is useful to identify and understand your personal barriers to following the different recommendations in the book. Make a list of strategies from this book or the DOZe app that would be most relevant and helpful for you, but that, for whatever reason, you have not been able to implement consistently. Now that you have a list of the recommendations regarding possible causes of your problems, write down possibilities for what got in the way. Write uncensored and explore every possible reason. Once you have identified some likely culprit "barriers," write uncensored any possible solutions to this problem. You may find it useful to use the Troubleshooting Barriers Worksheet (which you can download at http://www.newharbinger.com/44383). For example, you may find that removing wakeful activities from your bedroom is difficult because it would force you to go to the more common areas in your living space that may not give you the privacy you desire. This is a tricky issue that might require numerous possible solutions to test out until you find one that works.

EXAMINE YOUR VALUES

Sometimes you might discover that your dislike of getting rid of behaviors you value outweighs your dislike of your sleep problem. Examining what you value may help you discover whether this is why behavior change is difficult. Rate how much you value each of the following behaviors (0 = not at all important to me; 5 = very important to me):

- Sleeping in on the weekend.

- Being spontaneous in deciding when to get into and out of bed.

- Using caffeine and other sleep-interfering substances.

- Doing wakeful activities in bed, such as streaming, reading, or gaming.

- Spending a lot of time in your room.

- Staying up late.

- Using the *snooze* feature on your alarm.

How high is your total score? If it is high or if there are a few items that are rated highly, that may put you at odds with certain aspects of this treatment. This is normal. It sometimes helps to think about the cost and benefits of making a change. Write out the costs of the behavior change. For example: "The cost of regulating my sleep schedule is that I will feel like I can't be spontaneous. I want to be able to sleep in when I need to, and I like to hit the snooze button at least once before getting up." Now write out the benefits: "I will sleep better, and I am having trouble getting through the school day because I feel so bad. Having a more regular schedule will help my mood and alertness too. I might be able to make a minor change to my schedule and still experience benefits." Now look at the cost and benefits side by side. This will allow you to make a decision that is consistent with your values. It is okay if you decide not to make a behavior change right now, or if you decide to make a more modest change and evaluate whether it helps (for example, using the snooze button only once). Even if your values are at odds with the treatment right now, you may feel differently a week from now, in which case you can revisit whether you want to work on your sleep problem.

ENLISTING THE HELP OF OTHERS

Parents, teachers, counselors, and friends are often useful in helping with aspects of this treatment. That said, one complaint young adults often have is that they feel "preached at" or "judged" if they ask for help in making a change. It is important to make a specific request about what it is that you would like.

Broad request: "Can you help me? I'm trying to sleep better."

Specific request: "If you notice I am not up by 8 a.m. on weekdays, could you please knock on my door and then turn on my light?"

Which of these requests is more likely to be met with advice? You may not be able to stop criticism or unwanted advice, but broad or vague requests tend to elicit more of that than a very specific request. It's better to be very specific. If the person is not helpful, thank them and try someone else.

ADVICE FOR PARENTS, TEACHERS, AND COUNSELORS HELPING YOUNG ADULTS WITH THIS TREATMENT

We want our children (or students, or patients) to sleep better. We see that it is important and may be causing problems, so there can be a tendency to become frustrated and desperate in dealing with young adults, which often results in resistance and no behavior change. We have to acknowledge when our communication style isn't working, and be open to other ways of communicating that may help move young adults toward better sleep goals.

Be empathetic: They have a sleep problem and want support, not scorn, catastrophizing, or criticism.

Wait for an invitation: Wait for your offer of help to be accepted. Until it is, your role should be limited to sympathetic support.

If you are invited in, here are some communication tips that make it more likely that you will form a productive alliance.

Reflect: Restate what they say so that it is clear that you are listening. This is a tough one because they may say something that we wish they weren't thinking. "Sounds like you find it hard to turn your phone off when it feels like you are going to miss out on something."

Acknowledge that it is their choice: Once invited in, openly support their free will. Otherwise, they may feel like they need to dig in and reject any advice you provide. If you place an acknowledgement of their situation adjacent to their motivation for wanting change, they are more likely to want to make a change, instead of feeling like they are being pressured to make the change. "It's up to you if you want to make changes, but I am hearing that this sleep problem is really bothering you right now."

Support steps toward a plan: If they are frustrated that they haven't been able to meet their goal, reflect that fact back to them nonjudgmentally so they can see the two sides. "So you believe that turning off your phone is the key to sleeping better and going to bed earlier, but it has been tough to do this because you might miss out on something. Do I have that right?"

If they ask you to help with a plan, ask them questions so that they are constructing the plan. Your questions can help fine-tune the plan to make it achievable. Support any concrete step toward a positive change, even if it doesn't go as far as you would like. For example, if your teen makes a plan to turn off notifications but to leave the phone in their room "in case" they need to check, you could say: "That sounds like a good start. At least you won't be woken up by a notification. I guess if you find yourself looking at your phone throughout the night, you can decide if you need to go one step further to sleep better."

The way we communicate with someone attempting to make a behavioral change can make all the difference in whether we are helping or creating a situation in which the young adult feels committed to resisting any advice.

IS IT TIME TO SEE A SLEEP SPECIALIST?

It is always possible that some other sleep problem accounts for your sleep complaint. For example, if you have misidentified your sleep problem as insomnia when it is actually due to sleep apnea, following the advice in previous chapters will *not* help you and it is vital to get treatment for the apnea. Below are some signs of sleep problems that require further consultation with your family doctor.

CHECK FOR SIGNS OF OTHER SLEEP PROBLEMS

Signs of Sleep Apnea

Obstructive sleep apnea is a sleep-related breathing disorder that can cause a number of serious illnesses and can severely affect how you function during the daytime. Many people, including some doctors, assume that sleep apnea occurs mainly to middle-aged, overweight men, but sleep apnea can also strike children, young adults, women, and older adults. Because of all the problems it causes, it is important to assess for the signs of this disorder.

1. Do you snore loudly (for example, could someone hear you snore through a closed door? Is it as loud as a conversation?) and persistently (not just when you have an allergy flare-up or a cold)?

2. Are you a restless sleeper?

3. Do you fall asleep during the day?

4. Have you started having bed-wetting accidents, or do you have to get up to go to the bathroom more than twice a night?

5. Has anyone ever seen you stop breathing in your sleep, or heard you gasp, snort, or choke in your sleep?

6. There are also general risk factors for apnea to consider: Are you significantly overweight? Have other people in your family been diagnosed as having obstructive sleep apnea? Do you have an enlarged tongue or any problems with the nose or mouth that could constrict your airway?

If you said yes to two or more of these questions, it is important to raise the issue with your doctor. If your doctor has a belief that sleep apnea doesn't occur in teens, it is important to ask your parents to pursue an appointment with a sleep specialist. Teens and young adults *can* have sleep apnea and can get misdiagnosed as having attention deficit hyperactivity disorder or emotional problems because of the daytime problems this disorder can cause. Treatments can include surgery to correct whatever is blocking the airway (for example, having tonsils removed), a dental appliance to be worn at night, or delivering air via a mask to keep the airway open.

Signs of Narcolepsy

Narcolepsy is a disorder that typically emerges during adolescence. It is a neurological disorder characterized by rapid eye movement (REM) sleep occurring during the day. This disorder can create potentially unsafe situations, and it has a very large negative impact on your quality of life if left untreated. Here are some signs to watch for:

1. Do you struggle to stay awake during the day?

2. Do you fall asleep suddenly and involuntarily during the day, even in unusual places and at unusual times, as if it were a sleep "attack"?

3. Do you experience sudden muscle weakness for several seconds while awake? The muscle weakness may include only your knees buckling, but there can also be more muscle groups involved, including those of the face, neck, and shoulders, which may cause the body to collapse and fall. These episodes typically occur in response to emotions such as being startled, laughing, or crying.

4. Do you wake up paralyzed except for your eyes, for seconds or minutes at a time? This can happen for other reasons, especially if you are sleep-deprived, so it is not necessarily suggestive of narcolepsy.

5. Do you have strange visual hallucinations (such as strange moving patterns on the wall) when waking up or falling asleep?

Other Possible Signs for Concern

1. Struggling to stay awake during the day.

2. Sleep walking.

3. Eating while asleep.

4. Persistent nightmares.

5. Waking up in a panic.

6. People telling you that you wake up terrified or confused but you don't remember it.

7. Anything else that seems unusual.

If you experience any of these problems, it is worth a discussion with your doctor. There are many excellent doctors without much training in the sleep disorders of young adults, so if you are not satisfied with your doctor's response, you and your parents can discuss whether a consultation with a sleep specialist would be helpful. In North America, the American Academy of Sleep Medicine and the Canadian Sleep Society maintain lists of sleep specialty providers. Links to these and other resources are provided in the "Suggested Readings and Resources," downloadable at http://www.new harbinger.com/44383.

Summary

- Use the Sleep Tracker to evaluate whether you still have sleep problems.

- Use the Sleep Tracker to evaluate whether you are implementing the recommended changes.

- Troubleshoot difficulties by analyzing what's wrong and think of new solutions to test.

- Consider enlisting the help of someone by making a specific request.

- It may be that you value keeping the behavior in place more than you value getting rid of the sleep problem, and that is okay. This may change in the future.

- If you are unhappy with the results, or notice signs of another sleep disorder, talk to your doctor.

Colleen E. Carney, PhD, is associate professor and director of the Sleep and Depression Laboratory at Ryerson University in Toronto, ON, Canada. She was a National Sleep Foundation Pickwick Fellow at Duke University Medical Center, where she was on faculty, and she founded the Comorbid Insomnia Clinic at the Duke Insomnia and Sleep Research Program. Carney is well known for her publications in the area of insomnia and its relation to other disorders, most notably, depression, anxiety, and pain. She has made numerous presentations at national research conferences, including the Association for Behavioral and Cognitive Therapies (ABCT) and the Association for Professional Sleep Societies (APSS). She is president of the ABCT's Behavioral Sleep Medicine Special Interest Group for insomnia and other sleep disorders. Carney conducted research, funded by the National Institute of Mental Health, on treating insomnia in people with depression; and is currently conducting research, funded by the Canadian Institutes of Health Research, on treating the sleep problems of teens and young adults to help with mental health problems.

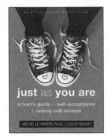
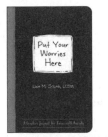
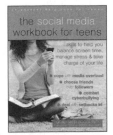
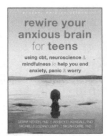
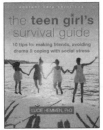
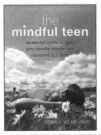

Register your **new harbinger** titles for additional benefits!

When you register your **new harbinger** title—purchased in any format, from any source—you get access to benefits like the following:

- Downloadable accessories like printable worksheets and extra content

- Instructional videos and audio files

- Information about updates, corrections, and new editions

Not every title has accessories, but we're adding new material all the time.

Access free accessories in 3 easy steps:

1. Sign in at NewHarbinger.com (or **register** to create an account).

2. Click on **register a book**. Search for your title and click the **register** button when it appears.

3. Click on the **book cover or title** to go to its details page. Click on **accessories** to view and access files.

That's all there is to it!

If you need help, visit:

NewHarbinger.com/accessories

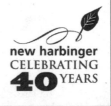

new harbinger
CELEBRATING
40 YEARS